Coping wi

Shirley Trickett trained as a nurse   d
teacher. She is the author of *Irritab._____ .sis*
(Thorsons 1987), *Coping with Anxiety and Depression, Coping Successfully
with Panic Attacks* and *Coping with Headaches* (all Sheldon Press). In 1987
she won a Whitbread Community Care Award.

Overcoming Common Problems Series

Selected titles

A full list of titles is available from Sheldon Press,
36 Causton Street, London SW1P 4ST, and on our website at
www.sheldonpress.co.uk

Overcoming Common Problems

Coping with Candida
Are yeast infections draining your energy?

SHIRLEY TRICKETT

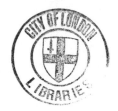

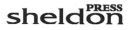

First published in Great Britain in 1994

Sheldon Press
36 Causton Street
London SW1P 4ST

Second edition published 2007

British Library Cataloguing-in-Publication Data

A catalogue record for this book is available from the British Library

ISBN 978-1-84709-012-6

1 3 5 7 9 10 8 6 4 2

Typeset by Fakenham Photosetting Ltd, Fakenham, Norfolk
Printed and bound in Great Britain by Ashford Colour Press

Contents

With love and gratitude for my friend Will Day,
my Australian 'kindred spirit'

Introduction

This book was first published in 1994. The question must be asked as to why there should be a need for a self-help book on fungal infections; they have been around for thousands of years. The planet changes, the human immune system changes, but, unfortunately, rigid medical attitudes do not change. What is not taught in medical schools takes at least three generations to be accepted in general medical practice. The purpose of this book is to bring information to those who suffer from fungal infections, mainly *candida albicans*. The problems range from repeated minor infections to chronic systemic candidiasis. As will be explained later, this is not a life-threatening condition, except where there is already serious illness. Millions of people worldwide are 'sick and tired of being tired and sick', when if their symptoms were recognized they could be treated and could feel well.

The problem in general practice

Minor conditions such as thrush and skin and nail infections will be treated in the doctor's surgery. If the initial infection clears up, that is fine; but so often anti-fungal medication is not taken for long enough and the infection recurs. Repeated infections do not seem to be questioned. More short-term prescriptions follow without thought about what is happening in the patient's immune system. Doctors trained in clinical nutrition or those with an interest in complementary medicine have a better understanding of the problem and usually use longer-term, non-drug anti-fungal treatments. These are much less toxic, and they also educate the sufferer on the importance of diet and boosting the immune system.

It is very rare for a GP to mention diet or probiotics (these will be discussed later), or for chronic candidiasis to be considered. Patients may well be sent for tests for other conditions, which come back negative. They may then be told they are 'just depressed', or, sadly, treated as a hypochondriacs. The illness caused by the spread through the body of the yeast *candida albicans*, and (to a much lesser degree) *candida tropicalis, parapsilosis, giulbrata* and *giulliermondii*, can take its place among the many medical conditions that, although they have been around for decades, have to become rampant before they are recognized by mainstream medicine.

Candida joins the queue alongside ME, fibromyalgia and other conditions that are destroying the lives of millions of people worldwide. It seems that what does not appear in the medical school curriculum does not exist. Systemic candida does indeed exist and is here to stay until it is recognized in the GP's surgery, the first place a sick person goes for help.

Resistance to change

Change has to be accepted. Why is it so much easier for scientists to acknowledge environmental damage than to see that the human organism, particularly the immune system, is also changing? It cannot cope with the toxic load of modern living. We are paying the price for the overuse use of antibiotics, steroids and hormones. The immune system cannot cope. 'New' illnesses can no longer be ignored. As long ago as 1970 Japanese researcher Dr Inata wrote his first article on candida. Pioneer doctors Crook and Truss wrote their books *The Yeast Connection* (1982) and *The Missing Diagnosis* (1983).

Choosing this book

You could have picked up this book thinking 'What on earth is candida?', or you might have chosen it because you suffer from repeated attacks of thrush and know that this is the organism responsible for the condition. Or it might be that you have battled for years with chronic problems and are looking for answers as to why your 'irritable bowel' does not respond to conventional treatment, why you have food and chemical intolerances, why you suffer chronic fatigue, why you cannot lose weight on a calorie-controlled diet, why you crave sweet or yeasty foods, why you have thrush before every period, why your PMS is getting worse, or why you have mood swings and other psychological symptoms. These are all problems that can be due to an overgrowth of candida in the bowel.

It is true that many of the above problems have their origin in conditions other than candida and it would be unwise to act hastily before you have consulted your doctor. If on the other hand your symptoms have been investigated and you have not had satisfactory answers then it would be worthwhile looking at the list of predisposing factors (particularly if you have been on long-term antibiotics).

What is candida?

Candida is a yeast which is normally present in the bowel. It feeds on the simple carbohydrates we eat such as sugar, bread, biscuits and cakes, and fermented foods such as cheese, alcohol and vinegar. If the immune system is healthy the growth of the candida can be kept under control; if it is not healthy, having been weakened by stress, conditions such as ME, fibromyalgia, cancer, AIDS, or any illness that depresses the immune system, candida can proliferate to such an extent that it can cause as many problems as the original illness. Prescribed drugs such as antibiotics, chemotherapy or steroids are major causes of candida overgrowth. Also, if resistance is low through poor nutrition, excessive alcohol, stress, illness or pollution, then the yeast can grow to such an extent that it interferes with normal body chemistry and can cause widespread baffling symptoms.

Is candida just the 'in thing' to have?

Sceptics have said of people with chronic candida problems that they read too many magazine health articles; that people love lists of symptoms; that candida is just the malady of the moment – a whitewash for hypochondrias and neurotic symptoms. Perhaps those who are not willing to look at the possibility of candida overgrowth causing chronic health problems should look at the alarming increase of anti-yeast prescriptions over recent years; they might ask themselves why, if the problem does not exist, there is a need for candida helplines and support groups and, most important, why these patients lose all their 'neurotic' symptoms when they are correctly diagnosed and receive the appropriate treatment – anti-fungal preparations – and make dietary adjustments.

The content of this book

This book describes what an overgrowth of candida can do to the body: how it can produce conditions that range from minor irritations to severe debilitating physical and psychological illness. It discusses the causal factors and who is most likely to be at risk. It also highlights why so many people are affected and why there is a division of medical opinion on the subject. Importantly, from your point of view, the following pages should enable you to decide whether your long-investigated symptoms arise from an overgrowth of fungus and, if so, happily, what you can safely do about it. It seeks not only to give clear suggestions on how to control candida with safe anti-fungal preparations, diet and nutritional supplements, but also shows you how to keep your digestive tract clean and build up your immune system to prevent further attacks. My frustration is that the conventional medical approach only leaves time, for example, to prescribe Canestan pessaries to a woman who has repeated thrush before her period without ever attempting to educate her on why this is happening and how to prevent further infections.

Light on a dreary subject

A book on bloated, aching abdomens, swollen sore penises and unpleasant discharges from the vagina cannot exactly be described as light reading, but I trust you will find these pages revealing and optimistic. I also anticipate that you will take heart from the case histories of people whose illness has previously defied diagnosis who have finally, through their own searching, overcome years of physical or psychological problems. It is quite an ascent from being a helpless 'thick-file' patient to being a healthy human being with a good knowledge of how to stay that way.

The good news

As I start to write this book the words of my old Sister Tutor ring in my ears: 'First reassure the patient'. So I am trying to be an obedient – if somewhat ancient – student nurse when I say that no matter how closely you identify your symptoms with the more severe form of the condition described in this book (systemic candidiasis), and although the list of symptoms looks awesome, do not be alarmed: treatment is effective and you can be well again.

How long will it take?

For long-term sufferers I do not pretend that this book offers overnight cures. Several months of treatment might be necessary. Taking a long, hard look at how you are living your life and why you are hurting yourself might also be an important part of the treatment for you. Some people find the physical treatments, such as diet and supplements, relatively easy, but resist change of lifestyle, giving up destructive thought patterns and establishing a relationship with their 'inner child'. I believe that total health depends on the harmony of body, mind and spirit. Discord causes tension and renders the body susceptible to illness of all kinds.

Using your recovery time to the full

Tackling any health problem can be a time for personal growth, a time to stop rushing around, a time to make a space in which you can not only understand your needs and make them known to those around you, but also lovingly meet those needs. Your first duty is to yourself.

1

The candida question

I must say at the outset that although I am a teacher of self-help and work with complementary medicine, I still have one foot in the other camp and stress that self-diagnosis is dangerous. You must describe your symptoms to your doctor before you embark on self-help programmes.

Candida albicans (thrush): why write a book on an organism that is normally present in the gut of every individual soon after birth, a yeast commonly thought to be responsible for little more (except in severely ill people) than infections of the mouth, vagina and irritating skin rashes? The answer is that twenty-first-century living – the environment, prescribed drugs (including the pill), street drugs, the ever-increasing consumption of alcohol, junk food, additives, sugar, and the pace of modern living – is slowly changing the human immune system. A healthy gut is an important part of the immune system. It needs to be a balanced ecological system, an environment where there are enough useful bacteria to attack harmful bacteria and keep the growth of fungus (yeasts) at bay, rather like keeping the weeds in the garden under control.

What an overgrowth of candida can do

When candida or other harmful yeasts rule, the sites in the bowel where substances called enzymes live, which are necessary for the breakdown of the food we eat, become blocked. This results in poor digestion, food intolerances, bloating, and altered bowel habits. An overgrowth in the colon can also inhibit the absorption of essential nutrients. That is why so many people on perfectly adequate diets can have vitamin and mineral deficiencies. In addition, the vitamins normally manufactured in the bowel cannot be produced when the colon is in this state, and thus the problem is compounded.

When there is a proliferation of candida it can change from its simple form, which looks like a microscopic fried egg, to a complicated invasive form which grows tentacles which are able to penetrate the bowel wall. This not only allows the toxins (which include alcohol) produced by the candida to circulate, but also gives the organism transport to other parts of the body where infections can arise, resulting in any of the following symptoms.

Physical symptoms

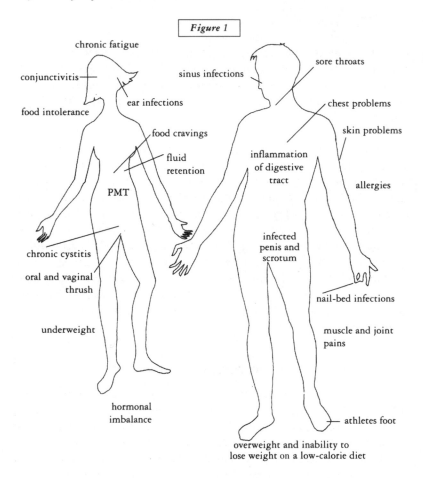

Figure 1

chronic fatigue

conjunctivitis

food intolerance

sinus infections

ear infections

food cravings

fluid retention

PMT

chronic cystitis

oral and vaginal thrush

underweight

hormonal imbalance

sore throats

chest problems

skin problems

inflammation of digestive tract

allergies

infected penis and scrotum

nail-bed infections

muscle and joint pains

athletes foot

overweight and inability to lose weight on a low-calorie diet

Brain symptoms

The toxins from the candida can cause severe psychological symptoms such as agitation, mood swings, anxiety, insomnia and depression.

The medical argument

Because of general lack of awareness on this subject and possibly the diversity of the symptoms, which could be interpreted as hypochondriasis, the long-term sufferer often has endless tests without the condition being diagnosed. If treatment is given, it is usually in the form of antibiotics, which aggravate the symptoms; or alternatively the patient is told 'This is only your nerves – why not take a holiday?'

My experience of working in the community for over 25 years leads me to believe that any condition that the average doctor has not met in medical school, in his or her mind does not exist. In saying that, please do not think I am without respect for the medical profession; I have met many doctors who are open and don't let the white coat (and the fear) cloak their own intuitive knowledge, who can let their patients express fully their intuitive feelings about their own bodies before they reach for the prescription pad. Again, I am not anti-drug, but very much against some of the lethal pharmacological cocktails so commonly prescribed in these 'pills-for-all-ills' days. I am also concerned by the endless repeat prescriptions for 'safe' drugs, such as medication for gastric ulcers. I have seen too many prescribed-drug damaged people, and, in this case, many who now face their doctors with chronic conditions, including candidiasis, which have resulted directly from their drug treatment. Not that drugs are the only cause of the candida problem; this will become clearer as you read.

What is fungus?

The fungi family includes moulds, mushrooms, yeasts and rusts. They are simple plants which lack chlorophyll, and are parasitic, living off live matter, or saprophytic, living off dead matter.

Yeasts are single-cell organisms that reproduce by budding (the formation of a small outgrowth that grows and breaks off) and possess enzymes capable of converting sugar into ethanol (alcohol). This process, called 'fermentation', causes the release of carbon dioxide. In bread-making the dough 'rises' because of this gas. Other products of fermentation are citric acid, oxalic acid, and butyric acid (see page 43). These are formed by certain bacteria.

Fungus is a mass of fine threads from which branches grow upwards. Spores are released from spore cases at the end of each branch. These grow into a new individual and can be carried by the wind. Fungi are all around us: in our bodies, in the soil and in the air. Some are helpful to us for digestion, baking, brewing and producing antibiotics; others are responsible for diseases in humans, animals and plants.

Causes – the likely candidates

It has been said that there is an increase in fungal infections in the population generally because of modern living. Predisposing factors that make some people particularly vulnerable are listed below:

- Any debilitating illness that weakens the immune system, such as flu, pneumonia, cancer or AIDS. (When the body already has more work than it can cope with, it cannot be vigilant enough to keep harmful organisms in the gut under control. In addition, immunosuppressant drugs, often vital in life-threatening diseases, encourage the body to play host to candida and other fungi. Adequate nutrition and supplements can prevent fungal overgrowth in seriously ill patients and very much improve their prognosis and quality of life.)
- Frequent treatment with antibiotics in the present or past.
- Using the contraceptive pill.
- Taking some prescribed medication (or, more commonly, after withdrawal from); for example, steroids, ulcer drugs, tranquillizers and sleeping pills, long-term antacids.
- Malnutrition: lack of vitamins and minerals, high-refined carbohydrate diet, junk foods.
- Stress.
- Endocrine disorders, diabetes.
- Genetic inability to cope with candida or carbohydrate.
- Anaemia.
- After any surgery, particularly abdominal surgery.
- Bowel infections, gastroenteritis.
- Damage to the urinary tract – catheterization.
- Hormonal imbalance: the premenstrual phase, pregnancy, the menopause.
- Multiple pregnancies.
- Ill-treating the immune system: lack of exercise and fresh air, polluted working environment.
- All street drugs.
- Alcohol.
- Lack of hydrochloric acid.
- Infection from sexual partner.
- A history of:
  - repeated bacterial infections

- hyperactivity as a child
- allergies
- swollen painful joints for no apparent cause
- oral thrush
- mouth ulcers
- chronic catarrh
- erratic vision: spots before eyes
- vaginal thrush, vulval itching
- itchy rectum or anus
- cystitis-like symptoms
- severe PMS
- unexplained mild raises in temperature
- jock itch
- athlete's foot, ringworm, psoriasis, nail-bed infections (a different organism but often associated with candida), acne
- craving for sweet or yeast-containing foods
- feeling worse after refined carbohydrates, alcohol, cheese, marmite, citrus juice, vitamin B or vitamin C tablets, soft drinks containing citric acid
- associating abdominal distension, breathing problems or any other symptoms with proximity to some chemicals
- wind, bloating, cramps, constipation, diarrhoea
- being weather-sensitive, worse in humid or wet weather
- feeling worse in musty or mouldy places
- irritability, confused thinking, poor memory, being 'spaced out', feeling drunk without alcohol, depression.

This chapter has given enough details for you to decide whether or not candida could be your problem. It is not an invitation to self-diagnose, but an opportunity for people whose symptoms have been investigated by a doctor to look for other avenues of help. People who have either been told that there is no apparent reason for their problems, or that it is 'just their nerves'.

Is it only candida that causes problems?

No. The fungi that cause infections are too numerous to mention but for the purposes of this book the term fungus will be used except where the yeast *Candida albicans* is known to be the definite culprit. If the body is weakened by an overgrowth of candida in the bowel, other fungi can intrude and the virulence of some of the harmful bacteria can also be increased.

What can I do to cope with fungal infections?

1 Kill the fungus.
2 Stop feeding it.
3 Clean the colon.
4 Replace the good bacteria in the gut – use probiotics.
5 Boost the immune system, with nutritional supplements, and by taking care of general health.

We shall be looking further at each of these later in the book.

2

Common fungal problems

Oral candida

This is a common infection. Anyone can get it but some people are more at risk than others. These include:

- Infants, who can be infected in the birth canal, from breast or bottle feeding, from dummies or kissing.
- Those in whom the environment of the mouth is not normal, for example people on drugs that cause a dry mouth, or those with injuries to the mouth such as from dentures rubbing, trauma or surgery.
- Diabetics, because high blood sugar levels feed candida.
- The elderly, where mouth hygiene and nutrition are often poor. Anaemia and B12 deficiency encourage candida.

The overuse of bacterial mouthwashes, taking antibiotics, steroids, ulcer drugs, chemotherapy, overuse of antacids (candida thrives in an acid environment), after withdrawal from tranquillizers, sleeping pills or antidepressant drugs can all be contributory factors. Close contact with an infected partner can put a person at risk from infection. A person might not be aware of the infection until it is noticed by a dentist, or until a partner complains about bad breath.

A severe infection

This is characterized by a furred tongue which has a white/greyish appearance. The insides of the cheeks, the gums, the palate and the throat can be covered with a white coating, which can be scraped off to reveal an inflamed area which sometimes bleeds. Blisters and ulcers can also be present.

Occasionally the white coating does not appear and the tongue can be smooth, and very red. In both cases a burning sensation and soreness can make eating painful. Opening the mouth is difficult if the infection spreads to the corners of the mouth. This is more common in the elderly and severely ill.

Prevention

Be strict about dental hygiene. You can gently brush your tongue or use a tongue scraper. Keep your toothbrush separate from those of other family members, change it regularly and disinfect it with a solution of Citricidal or tea tree oil (see also citricidal toothpaste, page 72). These can also be used as a mouthwash, as long as you use them away from the times when you take the pastilles, gel or suspension you have been given by the doctor. Avoid kissing. If you use an asthma inhaler rinse your mouth after every dose. Sip water regularly if you are on a drug that gives you a dry mouth. Your mouth might taste unpleasant. Resist the urge to suck sweets.

Repeated attacks

An odd infection is of no consequence but if you have repeated attacks there could be an underlying reason why this is happening, such as anaemia, or if you are diabetic that your blood sugar levels are too high. It could also be a warning that there is an overgrowth of candida in the bowel and you have, or are developing, systemic candidiasis.

Treatment

The drugs commonly used to treat oral candida are Amphotericin and Nystatin. These take the form of local treatment – they are not absorbed from the gastrointestinal tract – and consist of anti-fungal pastilles, suspension or gel. Treatment is usually for seven days but should be continued for two days after the symptoms have cleared. The suspension should be held in the mouth for as long as possible. Both this and the gel can be applied to dentures, but remove dentures and place in dental cleaning solution before sucking pastilles. If local treatment does not clear the infection, oral medication such as Fluconazole is needed.

People with severe illnesses, or those on drugs known to cause fungal problems, will have no trouble getting systemic treatment, but if you do not have a serious recognizable condition this could be difficult. As has been said, many GPs have little understanding of chronic candidiasis, and you might only be offered more topical treatment. If this is so it would be sensible to seek alternative help for the problem. This is discussed later.

Oesophagitis

Fungus is the main cause of inflammation of the oesophagus. It can occur as a follow-on from oral thrush or appear in isolation. It can also be a sign of a systemic fungal infection.

The area is covered with a white coating, which can be scraped off to reveal inflamed tissue. The symptoms are uncomfortable and if severe (usually in very ill people) swallowing can be painful and eating difficult. There can be pain behind the breastbone and a burning feeling which can be mistaken for heartburn. These symptoms are also experienced if there is an overgrowth of candida in the stomach together with nausea and loss of appetite.

This is not surprising. I once saw a stomach X-ray of a person with this problem. The candida looked like a large ball of cotton wool. After two weeks of treatment the second X-ray was completely normal. A light, liquid alkaline diet, such as soup, is recommended. Alkaline foods are listed in *Food Combining for Health* by Doris Grant and Jean Joice (see Further reading). Treatment is usually a suspension of an anti-fungal drug, covering the affected area. Care must be taken to see that the patient does not become dehydrated.

Fungal infections of the skin

Fungus is all around us so skin infections are common. An odd infection is likely to be caused by fungus entering damaged skin. Damp folds of skin, such as under the arms or in the groin (*intertrigo*) are the favourite areas, but the infection can appear anywhere. The appearance of the rash varies a great deal. It can be like sunburn, or red and scaly, sometimes with the addition of little pimples or larger pustules. It can also be under the skin and feel like small hard bumps. Itching can be intense. If scratching breaks the skin it can be complicated by a secondary bacterial infection.

Fungal skin infections can be mistaken for bacterial infections. Antibiotic treatment compounds the problem.

Rashes usually respond quite quickly to topical anti-fungals and giving the area as much air as possible. Sea bathing and a little sun often clear infections, in addition to medication. Tea tree oil (see page 78) stings a bit at first but is a very useful product. Not only is it a strong anti-fungal, it also helps itching because it has a slight local anaesthetic action.

It is important to:

- Finish the medication you are given, even if the skin is much improved.

- Wear cotton clothing and as little as possible indoors.
- Keep to your own towels and bed linen and wash these and clothing in water of no less than 60°C. If this is not possible disinfect laundry with Citricidal before washing (see page 72). Have your own kitchen towel or use kitchen rolls.
- Avoid steroid creams.
- Protect your partner by wearing nightwear that covers the infected area.

Repeated attacks

Don't dismiss these as just a nuisance and buy anti-fungal cream. Regular problems need treating from the inside. Look at the section on systemic candidiasis (Chapter 5).

Fungal nail infections

These are caused by a different fungus from skin infections, but respond to the same treatment. There are two types of nail infection which can affect fingers or feet.

Nail bed infection

The nail grows up from the cuticle discoloured and deformed and has more the appearance of horn. The feet can have a very unpleasant 'cheesy' smell.

Treatment

Long-term oral treatment is necessary, although creams are often also prescribed. This is usually for about three months or until the discoloured nail has completely grown out. People are often delighted to see clean, normal nail appearing as treatment progresses. Immersing the affected areas in water with added Citricidal or tea tree oil is useful. Instructions come with the products.

Tony

This young man noticed his big toenails became horny and discoloured after he had been taking long-term antibiotics for acne. When they began to discharge and smell unpleasant he saw his GP. He was prescribed two weeks on anti-fungal drugs and given a cream to rub into the cuticle. There was little improvement in those two weeks so he was given a three-month course of the drug orally. He was delighted to see normal nail growing in after several weeks, but as soon as the medication stopped the discharge returned, but the doctor was not happy about continuing the medication. Tony started to use Citricidal (see page 72) orally and locally. He had read about it in a magazine. He saw a homoeopath who gave him a diet sheet and what he described as 'little pills'. Nine months later his nails were white and smooth.

Nail border infection

Here the infected discoloured area is confined to the junction of the skin and nail. The rest of the nail looks normal. It can be that infection has entered through a whitlow. When the nail is pressed there is often a discharge of pus.

Treatment

This is the same as for nail bed infections, see above. If a finger is infected great care must be taken not to contaminate food, counter tops, the telephone, etc. Keep the finger covered when indoors, but when outside, where there is no danger of touching anything, it would benefit from the air. Keep your own nailbrush with your towel and have your own rubber gloves for household chores. You can buy thin cotton gloves to wear under rubber gloves.

Athlete's foot

This is an infection that can range from being just a mild irritation with peeling skin between the toes, to a painful condition that makes walking difficult. The sole of the foot can be red and swollen and sometimes blisters form. Cracks between the toes can also be painful. The skin between the fingers can be affected in the same way.

Remember to:

- Disinfect the shower base and bath after use.
- Get as much air to the feet or hands as possible. Wear sandals indoors and outdoors, weather permitting. If you have to wear shoes dust the insides with anti-fungal powder or use insoles and change frequently.
- Use a footbath twice daily.
- Change socks at least daily. These should be disinfected before washing and washed at a high temperature. Don't put them in the family laundry basket.
- Keep away from swimming pools or anywhere where you have to walk barefoot.

3

Women and candida

Thrush

Almost 30 years ago VD clinics reported the incidence of thrush in female patients examined to be as high as 28 per cent. Judging by the alarming increase in prescriptions for vaginal pessaries and creams, figures must be a great deal higher than that now. Repeated thrush infections – which often accompany cystitis – can make life a misery. Acute attacks are characterized by itching and soreness of the vagina and labia, with a creamy white discharge. This often has the appearance of cottage cheese. There is also a 'cheesy' odour.

An isolated attack of thrush which clears quickly with treatment is of no consequence. The fungus may gain entry because of some slight injury to vaginal tissue, either by vigorous sexual intercourse, a tampon, clothes chafing, or horse-riding. Long hot hours sitting travelling, particularly in nylon underwear or tight jeans, can also precipitate an attack. Increased sugar in the vaginal secretions in the premenstrual phase is the reason why there is often an attack at this time. If, however, you are getting regular infections, even if they do clear with local treatment, you should investigate why this is happening. Women with a reservoir of candida in the bowel, or deep in vaginal tissue, are more likely to suffer repeated attacks of thrush, although some have an atypical response, where there is no discharge but painful red swelling of the vulva, perineum and anus. The urethra can also be affected and passing urine can be painful.

If the condition is severe the skin can become cracked and bleed, or there can be hard creamy-coloured pustules. Long-term treatment is necessary for these symptoms (see the section on chronic candidiasis on page 23).

It is understandable that there is a higher incidence of thrush in women than in men. Oral contraceptives and hormonal influences must be the major reason for this. Candida in the bowel manufactures close on 50 chemicals; some of these are female hormones. The close proximity of the anus to the vagina (the area known as the perineum), and also the relatively short length of the urethra (the tube leading to the bladder), could account for women having more acute infections. Nevertheless, men are by no means immune from candidiasis and the numbers of sufferers are increasing. When an overgrowth is established in the bowel men suffer the same digestive problems, allergies, brain symptoms, and so on, as women.

Fungal cystitis

It is likely that candida can invade the bladder wall in the same way that it attacks the lining of the bowel or the vagina. I have seen hundreds of people here and abroad whose symptoms have failed to respond to antibiotics and whose urine analysis proved negative. Their symptoms did, however, finally respond to anti-fungal medication or to self-help anti-candida methods.

In the main, these people's symptoms were different from those of 'ordinary (bacterial) cystitis'. People prone to bacterial cystitis usually have isolated attacks causing pain, or burning on passing urine, which has an unpleasant smell and often contains pus or blood. Urgency and frequency are also features of bacterial cystitis. This symptom picture usually responds quite quickly to antibiotics, in contrast to fungal cystitis, which does not.

In fungal cystitis the symptoms tend to be less dramatic, more of a background discomfort in the bladder and the urethra which is made worse by citrus juices, alcohol, strong coffee, some soft drinks, and also by yeasty, sugary foods and some vitamin supplements, particularly vitamins C and B complex. It is true that a bladder inflamed by bacteria or viruses would also object to acid drinks, but it is unlikely that normal cystitis sufferers would be affected by eating bread or other foods normally included in their diet.

An important point to note is that urine specimens sent to microbiology departments are not tested for fungus without a special request. A typical general hospital might expect between 1 and 5 per cent of all urine specimens received for culture to contain yeasts. It is imagined that a large proportion of these specimens will be from patients with indwelling catheters or those who have been hospitalized for some serious condition requiring large doses of antibiotics. Few specimens will have come from GPs looking for fungal cystitis in their patients. If you identify your symptoms with those of fungal cystitis it would be wise to ask your doctor for a fungal test to be included in the investigations.

Fungal cystitis can be an infection in a single site, but it is more commonly seen in people who have fungal infections in other sites, for example in the gut, the vagina (thrush) or nail beds. An irritated bladder can also be a feature of food intolerance.

Proprietary medicines for cystitis

These can bring temporary relief to an inflamed bladder but should not be used for long periods. They work by making the urine alkaline and ease the inflammation in much the same way as an antacid soothes an irritated gastric lining. In both cases, it is unwise to use these preparations for prolonged periods because they upset the delicate acid–alkaline balance of the body and lead you into further troubles.

In the case of fungal cystitis a proprietory medicine may make you feel more comfortable, but since candida thrives in an acid medium it could eventually compound your problem. Some preparations contain citric acid.

Natural remedies for cystitis

Women are more prone to cystitis than men because they have a shorter urethra (tube leading from the bladder) and it is therefore easier for harmful organisms from the bowel to ascend into the bladder. The effect of cranberry juice on urinary tract infections has been discussed in many medical journals. There has been evidence for about 35 years that it can help to prevent infections. It works by preventing harmful bacteria, particularly *E.coli*, from attaching to the lining of the bladder.

There seems to be little doubt that cranberry juice can be extremely valuable in the prophylaxis (prevention) of urinary tract infections, especially for people with recurrence. It is probable that the relief of acute infection will always lie in the domain of antibiotics, but as well as causing side effects, they do diminish the body's own defences against the recurrence of the disease. Overall, urinary tract infections are such a major problem, notably of female health, that any effective addition to the armoury of the practitioner would be very welcome. One advantage of cranberry juice is that it cannot possibly do any harm – only good.

Cranberry juice is very popular in the United States. It can be found in delicatessens and supermarkets here, or even at the off-licence store where it is often stocked as a mixer for vodka. Cranberry juice preparations combined with acidophilus are available from BioCare (see Useful addresses).

Homoeopathy, herbs and essential oils are also used for the relief of cystitis.

At the slightest sign of discomfort in the bladder or urethra, drink as much water (preferably bottled) as you can and take a warm, shallow bath, if possible with ten drops of tea tree oil. This is available in most pharmacies. Sometimes a hot-water bottle on the lower back or abdomen helps. One teaspoonful of bicarbonate of soda in a pint of warm water often brings immediate relief of symptoms.

Even if there is no bacterial or fungal infection in the bladder it can become irritated by eating or drinking something you are intolerant to.

For more on the management of cystitis see Further reading at the back of this book.

Interstitial cystitis

This is a chronic inflammation of the bladder for which the cause is not clear. It is more frequent in women, but men can be affected and it can be misdiagnosed as non-bacterial prostatitis. It is a distressing condition and often severely affects the quality of life. The symptoms are urgency and frequency of passing urine and considerable pain in the pelvic area. 'Pinpoint bleeding' can occur but this is not seen in the urine and can only be detected with tests. Sufferers often notice that certain foods or drinks make the bladder and urethra feel 'raw'.

Tomatoes, fruit drinks (including cranberry juice), carbonated drinks, tea and coffee are often mentioned. Food intolerance could be a factor. Interstitial cystitis is a common symptom in fibromyalgia and ME. It has been reported that people diagnosed with this condition have been cured by taking anti-fungal drugs or supplements and following a sugar-free diet. See *The Candida-Related Complex – What Your Doctor Might be Missing* by Christine Winderlin with Keith Sehnert (see Further reading).

The premenstrual phase and candida

Any hormone disturbance can trigger an acute attack of thrush. Oral contraceptives have been shown to increase the vaginal glucose content by 50 to 80 per cent, thus providing a good food supply for the candida. In the premenstrual phase, during pregnancy and during steroid medication, the delicate acid–alkaline balance of the vaginal secretions is altered. This also encourages fungal growth.

The menopause and candida

During the menopause the vagina can lose its natural lubricant protection and become dry and cracked. This condition is called *atrophic vaginitis* and is caused by a decrease in the oestrogen levels.

When the tender mucous membrane of the vagina is torn, candida easily gains entry. Oestrogen creams are often prescribed for this, or a simple lubricant such as KY jelly. There are natural ways of increasing oestrogen levels. Boron, a substance found in vegetables and widely available as a food supplement in health food shops and from nutritional suppliers, has been found to be as effective as hormone replacement therapy. Cold bathing has also been found to raise oestrogen levels.

Look at the predisposing factors

- Have you got an overgrowth of thrush in the bowel?
- How stressed are you?
- Is your immune system working well?
- Do you have a high-refined carbohydrate, yeasty diet?
- Is your partner reinfecting you?

Medical treatment

Fluconazole: This is given as a single-dose capsule, often with a pessary. You should tell your doctor if you are on any other medication. The accompanying leaflet should be read very carefully.

This drug is on sale freely and many women continue to take it month after month. This is not recommended as it is a toxic drug. It can usually be used once, but after that it is better to continue with the safer non-drug anti-fungals. If you have had thrush more than twice in six months you should consult your doctor – although in saying that, the outcome might not be satisfactory. The long-term use of non-drug anti-fungals will be discussed later.

Clotrimazole cream: This is applied to the anogenital area three times daily, or as a single-dose pessary to be used at night.
Note: The effect on latex condoms and diaphragms are not yet known (British National Formulary).

Nystatin: This well-established drug works well locally or in the gut but is not suitable as a cream for chronic candidiasis. It is prescribed with an applicator or as pessaries to be used at night for at least two weeks.

Other vaginal infections

Gardnerella

This bacterium produces a greyish, frothy discharge that is often mistaken for thrush. If you have an infection that does not respond to anti-fungal treatment your doctor would usually prescribe the antibiotic Flagyl. Women with gardnerella who are prone to thrush may have both infections and would need both anti-fungal and anti-bacterial treatment.

Trichomonas vaginalis

This is caused by a parasite and is also often mistaken for thrush. The symptoms are similar but the discharge is usually darker and has a stronger smell. Flagyl is also prescribed for this condition. For non-drug preparations that are effective against both these infections see pages 70 and 72.

It is important to have long-term oral and local treatment since the infection can spread to the reproductive organs and cause pelvic pain.

Mothers, babies and candida
by Heather Welford

Candida can affect the early weeks and months of your baby's life, and bring pain and discomfort to one of motherhood's most pleasurable and rewarding experiences – breastfeeding. Candida on the nipples, and in the breast itself, can cause soreness, both during feeding and between feeds. It can be bad enough to make even the most dedicated and motivated breastfeeder turn to the bottle in desperation.

Babies, too, can get painful thrush infections on their bottoms and in their genital area. They can also have candida in the mouth, and this may mean it's painful to suck on a breast or bottle.

Thrush and feeding

When a breastfeeding mother complains of soreness, breastfeeding counsellors – mothers trained to help other mothers overcome breast-feeding problems – and professional lactation specialists are usually well aware that thrush could be the reason. But other advisers, including general practitioners, don't always know of the possibility. Mothers are sometimes told to stop feeding, or they are given creams and sprays that have no effect at all on the problem and may make it even worse.

Breastfeeding provides an ideal environment for candida to flourish, especially today in the West, where the breasts might be covered for most of the time with a hot, sweaty, synthetic fabric bra, maybe with a plastic-backed breast pad tucked inside for good measure.

In addition, many new mothers and babies are prescribed antibiotics, often because of a post-natal infection contracted in hospital. Doctors may also prescribe antibiotics as a routine preventive measure to mothers who have had a Caesarean section (more than 20 per cent of deliveries in the UK are now done this way). We've seen on page 4 that antibiotics can make candida conditions more likely.

If either you or your baby has thrush, breastfeeding can mean you pass it between you, backwards and forwards. Bottle-fed babies can get thrush in their mouths, too, as can babies who use a dummy.

Sore bottoms

Nappies are a relatively new invention, and they keep your baby's bottom warm and moist – again, ideal conditions for thrush. The thrush can affect the anus, the buttocks, the genitals and the top of the legs as well.

Symptoms

You may have sore, red, raw or itchy nipples. Sometimes the skin seems to flake away. The nipples are tender between feeds, and it can be very painful when the baby latches on.

However, if you've been sore from the very beginning, then poor positioning (with your baby sucking on the end of your nipple, instead of being well latched on to the breast) is a more likely cause than thrush. Yet you can get thrush on top of soreness caused by poor positioning; and if you're pretty sure your positioning is correct, and you still don't heal, suspect candida.

You may also get intense, stabbing or shooting pains in the breast, most acute when the baby is actually feeding or shortly afterwards. The pains tend to radiate out from the nipple and they may indicate that there is thrush in the breast milk ducts, or in the areas of the breast surrounding the ducts. It is possible to get these pains without any soreness on the nipples.

If your baby is affected by thrush, he or she may have a red, shiny patchy rash on the nappy area that doesn't go away with the usual remedies for nappy rash (exposing the bottom to the air, application of nappy rash cream, frequent nappy changes). The effects can be painful, and cause your baby some distress. That's not always the case, however; even quite dramatic-looking symptoms may not produce any soreness.

Oral thrush shows up as whitish deposits in your baby's mouth: on the tongue, the inside of the cheeks and the gums. A few babies show some reluctance to feed and cry when they suck. However, some babies with thrush don't show any symptoms; it is still sensible to assume that if you have it, and you're breastfeeding, then your baby has it too.

Treatment

- Discard all the teats and dummies you're using and buy new ones (sterilize them before use, of course). The same goes for any nipple shields. Shields are sometimes used to protect sore nipples, but they can make the problem worse not better, and they don't help the baby learn to latch on to the breast comfortably. Ask for help in positioning your baby on the breast so that you no longer need a shield.
- Wear a cotton bra, and change your breast pads often. Use non-plastic backed ones.
- See your doctor for anti-fungal medication, and insist on treatment for both you and your baby if you're breastfeeding. Really persistent candida can take a couple of weeks or more to clear, though you should see an improvement in a few days.
- Make sure you pay extra attention to family hygiene, with separate flannels and towels for each of you. Check other members of the family for candida, especially your sexual partner.
- If the thrush persists, check your diet (see page 80) and try some of the suggestions in Chapter 10.

Trisha

Trisha had been feeding baby Joshua for nine weeks, with no problems at all. Then she developed sore nipples. She described them as 'feeling raw'. Feeding was very painful, and her nipples were tender between feeds, too. Her doctor could give no explanation as to why she should develop the soreness after so many weeks of happy feeding, and prescribed some lanolin cream to soothe them. This, if anything, made the problem worse.

By chance, Trisha met a breastfeeding counsellor at a mutual friend's house. The counsellor said the problem could be caused by candida, and this seemed even more likely when Trisha reported a recent bout of vaginal thrush, which had started after a course of antibiotics for an infection.

Trisha's GP was willing to consider this diagnosis, and when Trisha went back he prescribed two separate anti-fungal preparations, one for her and one for Joshua. In a few days, the soreness had gone.

Heather Welford is a journalist and writer specializing in the areas of health, family interest, education and human interest.

4

Men and candida

Men going to the doctor with an overgrowth of intestinal candida (see page 23) are quite likely to be told they are suffering from diverticulosis or stress. Women are usually given the diagnosis of irritable bowel syndrome or perhaps ME. The chronic symptom picture in men is identical to women: the same physical symptoms as women except, of course, for the anatomical differences. In contrast, men often have alcohol-related candida and more chemical intolerances due to exposure in the workplace. They suffer just as much from digestive problems and food allergies – in fact more, because it often takes time to get them to understand the importance of diet. Weaning them away from the 'pie and pint' at lunchtime can be difficult.

Acute attacks

Infections around the genitals – 'jock itch' – are common. If the penis is inflamed it is likely to be combined with a bacterial infection. Thrush manifests in some men as non-specific urethritis (NSU). This infection needs medical attention since it can lead to a more serious condition called Reiter's syndrome, which consists of arthritis, urethritis, conjunctivitis and sometimes fever and rashes.

Contact dermatitis/candida

Contact dermatitis from buckles on belts, metal on jeans or from washing powders is often complicated by fungal infections and can be very persistent. If your efforts with anti-fungal creams fail, you should see your doctor.

Other causes

Because of raised glucose levels in the blood, diabetic men are prone to fungal infections. The perspiration can often smell 'yeasty'.

Heavy drinking not only feeds candida, it also depletes the immune system, disturbs blood glucose levels and prevents the absorption of nutrients which help to control fungal growth. Obvious symptoms of fungal problems, such as rashes, often do not appear until the person has stopped drinking. They are more commonly on the trunk and arms, and it could be more than coincidence that psoriasis often worsens during this period.

Infection of the penis (balanitis)

As can be imagined, this is a painful condition. There is often discharge and the skin can be cracked and tender. Passing urine may also be painful. Men can be infected through a partner who has thrush, but they can also carry the organism and be without symptoms and thus infect their partner. Medical treatment should be sought because of the danger of the infection spreading to the urinary tract. Strict hygiene is important. Underwear should be either soaked in Citricidal (see product instructions) or if possible washed at a high temperature. Often the infection is mild and is treated locally. It is important to carry on with treatment for at least two weeks after the symptoms have gone.

Mike

Mike, a 22-year-old student, described his life as complete misery when he came for help. His penis was so swollen and sore he found walking and even sitting in lectures difficult. In his room he wore only a long T-shirt and outdoors a loose tracksuit. It was impossible to wear jeans, his normal attire. He was also anxious, frustrated and depressed. He had no social life and was very worried about the future.

He had been seeing his doctor for several months and had initially been given antibiotics, and later anti-fungal drugs and cortisone cream. The anti-fungal treatment helped but within a few days of stopping treatment the symptoms returned. He was finally sent to a consultant at a 'Special Unit' (Department for Sexually Transmitted Disease) and was told he had both bacterial and fungal infections. He was given antibiotics and anti-fungal medication which were more effective than the anti-fungal treatment alone; but, again, once treatment stopped the symptoms returned.

It wasn't until he rang a candida counsellor, who asked about diet and food cravings, that he realized how much he craved cheese and marmite sandwiches and his daily pint of beer. He had reasoned that he ate the sandwiches, which were the mainstay of his diet, because they were convenient and economical; but then went on to say that if he ate out he always had one when he returned – the candida screaming for its favourite diet!

Because it was the least expensive, he chose the garlic method (see page 70) and made a half-hearted attempt at the candida diet. Two weeks later his condition had improved but he felt he would have to be stricter about the diet and take some of the suggested supplements. He tried acidophilus and yeast-free mineral and vitamin supplements. Four weeks later he was doing very well unless he reverted to his old habits.

5

Chronic or systemic candidiasis

Many people say, 'But I haven't had thrush, or ear problems, etc. for years.' If your body has been coping with an overgrowth of candida for some time it may no longer be responding with an acute infection. In effect it has become tolerant to the effects of the organism.

What is chronic or systemic candidiasis?

This is where the fungal infection is no longer local. It enters the bloodstream, as has been described (see page 1), by the tentacles of the organism puncturing the wall of the bowel and causing a bloodstream infection, which can then invade any tissue in the body. This is the common form of transmission. Occasionally it can occur during surgery when medical equipment becomes contaminated with candida.

The big problem

The infection can be anywhere in the body, and this is what causes the multitude of symptoms that are baffling to both patient and doctor. As has been said, it frequently adds to the patient's distress when, after other causes have been looked for, the 'It's only your nerves' diagnosis is so often made. Myalgic encephalomyelitis (ME) or fibromyalgia come up frequently as diagnoses, and this is not surprising since, as you will see later, the conditions have very similar symptoms and frequently coexist. If you complain of bloating, gas, diarrhoea or constipation you may be diagnosed (after investigations for more serious conditions prove negative) as having irritable bowel syndrome (IBS) or diverticulosis (see my book *The Irritable Bowel Syndrome and Diverticulosis* listed in Further reading). Food intolerances might also be suspected. If, however, your symptoms are diverse and include malfunctions of many of the systems of the body, as would be expected – if you are in a toxic state – it is unlikely that the appropriate diagnosis will be made, and even less likely that the correct treatment will be given.

Some symptoms of chronic candidiasis

- Feeling as though you have a 'chill' or flu, or recovering from flu most of the time.
- Fatigue.
- Headaches.
- Sore eyes.
- Continual low-grade ear, nose, throat problems and sinus problems.
- Oesophagitis.
- Tight chest.
- Sore mouth (not necessarily oral thrush), mouth ulcers.
- Muscle and joint pains.
- Digestion problems.
- Urinary problems.
- Severe PMS.
- Low libido.
- Depression – this can be severe (see page 2).
- Anxiety – panic attacks.
- Lack of concentration.
- Atypical reactions: no discharge but swelling and inflammation in the ano-genital area.

Some women with chronic candidiasis stop reacting with acute attacks, such as thrush. It is common for a chronic sufferer to say, 'Oh yes, I had attacks of thrush for years, but I don't get it now.' It is important for these women to look at these symptoms of chronic candidiasis.

Brain symptoms

Both sexes get brain symptoms. I do not call these psychological symptoms because they could be interpreted as problems caused by the distress of the physical symptoms. It is true that people often are in despair because they feel so ill and no cause can be found, but the main causes of the symptoms are biochemical – toxins from the candida and undigested proteins.

Women showing symptoms are often taken less seriously than men are. When women present to their doctors with symptoms of lethargy, anxiety, depression and so on, they may be told it's only their nerves, or their symptoms are attributed to their hormones: it's PMS, it's PMS extending over more of the month now that you are past 35, or it's the menopause. Undoubtedly part of the story can be the hormonal influence, but what about the rest? And why do these women fail to respond to tranquillizers, antidepressants and treatments for hormonal problems? Why do they recover only when they gain their own knowledge of candidiasis and act on it, or when they see a GP who understands where their symptoms are coming from? Misdiagnosis in women causes frustration, loss of confidence and in some instances, no doubt because of this, psychological problems are superimposed on the existing physiological manifestations of altered brain chemistry. Often when a woman feels improvement with anti-candida treatment there will be angry tears: 'I knew it was something in my body that was causing this; why did the doctor not listen to me?'

Systemic candidiasis – case histories

Raymond

I could not make sense of why I was so depressed. I had tried several antidepressants and they just made me feel worse. I had been with my partner for seven years and the relationship was good. My job was interesting and I had no financial problems. It was trying to help my partner that gave me the first clue. She gave up seeing the doctor and was buying Diflucan regularly but was still having problems with thrush. She claimed she had never had an attack before she met me. I found this hard to believe. I thought this was something that most women had. My ex-wife also had the problem.

I was buying a book for my mother's birthday when I saw a book on candida. I stood reading it in the shop for some time before I bought it. I was fascinated. Here was a complete picture of me, not just the depression, but the nausea, bloated abdomen, sinus problems and all the things my brother, a doctor, had laughed off as the 'male menopause'.

My partner felt the book made sense and we decided to go to London to see a doctor mentioned in the book. We had blood tests, were given anti-fungal drugs, and a diet sheet. My partner's symptoms cleared quite quickly, but I admit that she was much better at keeping to the diet.

After a month we were both given olive leaf extract instead of the drug. My partner did not have any problems with this but at first it made me feel queasy. I lost weight, which was needed. I was also told I must wear a condom to avoid reinfecting my partner.

It was hard for me to keep going because it was several weeks before I felt any better. After four months there was great improvement. Life felt worth living again. We are now both seeing a kinesiologist locally. It seems I also have other 'bugs' in my system to be dealt with. My doctor father would have called the man a quack, but who cares – we both find him very helpful.

My partner had to drag me away from researching on the internet to watch our favourite television programmes. I found the 'Mark Cobb' story and saw the parallels to my own illness. I feel confident to call it that now. It is an illness. I am not the type to be depressed and have all these strange symptoms all over. In retrospect, I think it started after I had had several courses of antibiotics for a septic foot. I trod on something on a beach in Spain and the skin kept 'breaking down'.

It is wonderful to be able to think clearly again and not want to sleep all the time. My gut does not swell up towards evening and I enjoy my food again. I feel that men with chronic candida problems might be particularly overlooked. I hope my story will be helpful to someone.

Lisa
Lisa had been ill for four years. After a period of prolonged stress she developed recurrent thrush, cystitis and severe premenstrual tension. These problems were all new to her and she became increasingly anxious and depressed. Her boyfriend and work colleagues began to lose patience with her. She feared her job could be in jeopardy. She had formerly enjoyed her work, but she became anxious, particularly when she was premenstrual, about going to the office because she reacted so explosively to events that would previously have caused her merely to feel mildly irritated. Visits to the doctor resulted in Canestan cream for the thrush or antibiotics for the cystitis. She was also urged to stop worrying.

Although she was losing weight, her abdomen grew alarmingly. She could not fasten her skirts. This coincided with altered bowel habits: bouts of constipation, then diarrhoea. Even when her stool was loose she felt 'windy' and never felt she had cleared her bowel. This was diagnosed as irritable bowel syndrome, which her doctor said was due to nerves. He suggested a high-fibre diet and again to stop worrying.

Two months later, when the next set of symptoms arrived, Lisa saw another doctor in the practice. She complained of swelling inside her nose, aching sinuses and a dry cough. She also mentioned that she felt ill when she ate certain foods and when she was near some chemicals. The symptoms associated with food intolerance were palpitations, restlessness, depression and nettlerash (hives). The effect of the chemical intolerance was a feeling of being 'spaced out', with headaches and an inability to concentrate. The smell in her new car and from the photo-copier at work seemed particularly to affect her.

She left the surgery with a prescription for a nasal spray and antihistamines. Both helped a little but she was still dissatisfied. She began reading health magazines and books and was delighted when she read a newspaper article by a woman who had an identical experience to her own. Armed with information on systemic fungal infections she saw yet another doctor in the practice. To her surprise and delight he agreed that this could be the problem and prescribed Nystatin. She also put herself on a strict anti-candida diet.

For the first three weeks she felt 'rough': new symptoms developed which she rightly assumed were just temporary. These were a slight temperature, feelings of confusion, and muscle and joint pains. As these cleared she made steady progress; all the symptoms she had suffered for years just seemed to drop away. Friends commented on her appearance: her face regained its normal contours (it had been bloated) and was free from the bumps under the skin and dryness that had contributed to her misery.

Lisa's story illustrates the diverse nature of chronic candidiasis, and how seriously the hormone balance can be upset.

Carol

At 39, Carol had successfully withdrawn from tranquillizers after taking them for ten years. Three months after withdrawal she complained of a bloated abdomen, a constant feeling of imminent cystitis and an ear infection. Her ear discharged a watery fluid, which dried into a crystalline deposit on her skin nearly to her chin. The skin became inflamed and had almost the appearance of a burn.

She was prescribed three different courses of antibiotics without any effect, before a laboratory test confirmed that she had a fungal infection. She was given anti-fungal ear drops and cream for her skin. The ear symptoms needed prolonged treatment but eventually cleared up. Her abdominal symptoms and urinary symptoms persisted until she went on an anti-candida diet.

Elizabeth

Elizabeth had a history of taking antibiotics: for ear infections as a child and as an adult for a kidney infection. For several years after the kidney infection she had feelings of impending cystitis, often associated with stress or eating certain foods.

After a particularly stressful period she noticed a slight dry rash on her body. It worsened over a period of ten days, until it separated into round red patches each about 1 cm across. It looked like cigarette burns and appeared on the trunk only, not on the limbs or her face. Itching was a problem especially when she was hot.

The doctor diagnosed *pityriasis rosacea* and said it was caused by an airborne virus that she could have picked up on a bus; there was no cure and it would clear up of its own accord within about three months. Elizabeth was horrified at the thought of having such a disfiguring, uncomfortable rash for so long and also realized it would prevent her from swimming or taking any exercise that would make her hot.

The name was the clue to the whole business. After her visit to the doctor she found out that her cousin had had the same symptoms but her doctor had diagnosed the rash as a fungal infection. She bought a book on candida and started on an anti-candida diet immediately. She was very strict about sugar (even fruit), bread and cheese, and not quite so strict with wine and diet Coke. Vegetables, fish, lamb and free-range, corn-fed eggs were the mainstay of her diet. Other red meats and battery eggs were avoided because antibiotics are included in the feed.

Elizabeth used essential oils in her daily bath – lavender and tea tree, three drops of each. Two drops of each oil were mixed with one dessert-spoonful of olive oil and applied to the rash twice daily. This was very helpful for the itching. She also had sun bed treatment every three or four days.

A telephone counselling session with a nutritionist resulted in her starting supplements. These included caprylic acid, superdophillus, and herbal tablets and psyllium husks as part of a bowel cleansing programme. She also drank Pau d'Arco anti-fungal herbal tea. For the first week or so after starting the diet, the rash got worse. After about ten days there was slight improvement, which was definite a few days later. After that she could see it clearing before her eyes; it seemed to retreat inwards, being most stubborn in the warmer places, around the armpits and stomach.

Three weeks after her first visit to the doctor she went back to show him the results. Her skin was almost perfect in a fraction of the time he had told her. He was astonished but did not show any interest in how she had cured herself. He was pleased, but just seemed to think it was a bit of unusual good luck.

Elizabeth's story illustrates how attacking fungal skin infections from inside as well as outside can achieve rapid results. Fungal skin problems need not be as dramatic as this; they can come and go, depending on how stressed you are or what you are eating.

Mavis

Mavis had suffered from sore fingers for years. The tips were tender and cracked, and when they were at their worst they would bleed. She had tried creams from the doctor and wearing gloves for housework but these measures did not help. She was elderly and on a low income, so she was advised to try simple things first, such as cutting down on sugar and tea and eliminating wheat altogether, substituting Ryvita for bread. She was encouraged to eat more vegetables and take one multimineral and one multivitamin tablet daily (both yeast-free). Three days after giving up bread she saw improvement and after a week her fingers had completely healed.

Mavis was delighted: she could knit, sew and do her housework without any problems. After three weeks she decided to try bread again to see what would happen. She had half a slice; the following day her fingers were inflamed and sore. She stayed wheat-free for three months, then found she could eat a scone or bread two to three times a week without problems.

It could be said that Mavis's sore fingers were due to a wheat allergy and not fungal infection. Experience has shown, however, that candida and allergy very often go together. In this instance it did not matter what the cause was: the simple suggestions cleared up a long-standing painful condition. It could be said that skin problems often seem to be a neglected area of medicine. Since they are not life-threatening and people are usually still mobile, they are often left to get on with them.

John

John's story shows that fungal problems can arise in people who are perfectly healthy, until they include something in their diet which causes the candida in the bowel to multiply.

John had an unbearably itchy rash around his anus, scrotum and up into his groin. He was losing sleep, becoming irritable and finding it impossible to sit still in meetings. His work was suffering because of poor concentration. Sitting in cold water was the only way he could ease the itching. The creams he had been given by the doctor worked to some extent but the effect did not last.

John's diet and lifestyle both seemed healthy: adequate exercise, lots of vegetables, salads, fruit and fish; he was a non-smoker who drank moderately at weekends only. All was revealed when he was asked about stress. He replied that things had been a bit hectic at work recently and that he was taking brewer's yeast tablets for extra B vitamins. A colleague had recommended them. It had not occurred to him that the onset of his symptoms might be associated with taking the tablets. He thought they were an old-fashioned, healthy addition to the diet and even if they did not actually improve things, at least they could not do him any harm.

In reflection John saw the connection: he started the tablets the week before a conference and slight itching had started the following week.

It had gradually become more severe and had continued to date. All he had to do to cure himself was to stop taking the tablets and drink lots of water. After only two days he was much improved; a week later his skin was back to normal.

6

Allergies and food intolerance

An allergic reaction is an inflammatory response by the body to a substance to which it is exposed, either by inhalation, ingestion or through contact with the skin. Common allergic responses are seen in asthma, nettlerash, hay fever and eczema. Extreme reactions to one or two foods mean that these have to be avoided for a lifetime. Symptoms can be severe, sometimes necessitating admission to hospital. They include itching, difficulty in breathing, swelling of the lips, tongue and throat, and nausea. Severe food allergy is a well-recognized medical condition. What is perhaps less well documented is sensitivity or intolerance to certain foods.

Food intolerance

This is also known as a masked or hidden allergy, and happens with foods that are eaten regularly. When they are stopped, cravings and other withdrawal symptoms can develop. Food intolerance is not well diagnosed, possibly because the symptoms can be vague and confused with other conditions, particularly psychological problems; the patient is often dismissed as neurotic. Symptoms look very much like those of candida overgrowth and the two conditions usually coexist. They are:

- flushing, sweating after meals
- foul taste in mouth, loss of taste
- sore mouth, mouth ulcers
- abnormal thirst
- asthma
- hives (nettlerash)
- inflamed digestive tract
- bloating
- continuous dull abdominal ache
- constipation
- diarrhoea
- flattened stool
- feeling of never having a complete bowel movement

- itching anus
- frequency of urine
- urgency of stool
- feeling of the brain being swollen
- irritability, outburst of rage
- feeling of being 'spaced out'
- anxiety or depression after eating certain foods
- chronic fatigue
- hyperactivity.

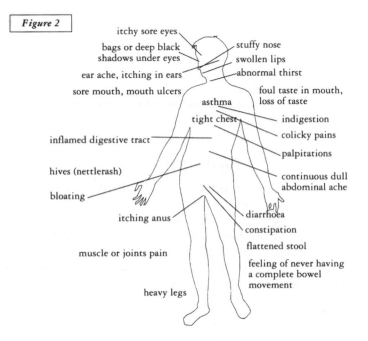

Figure 2

itchy sore eyes

bags or deep black shadows under eyes

ear ache, itching in ears

sore mouth, mouth ulcers

stuffy nose

swollen lips

abnormal thirst

foul taste in mouth, loss of taste

asthma

tight chest

inflamed digestive tract

hives (nettlerash)

bloating

itching anus

muscle or joints pain

heavy legs

indigestion

colicky pains

palpitations

continuous dull abdominal ache

diarrhoea

constipation

flattened stool

feeling of never having a complete bowel movement

Often these symptoms go on for years, with the sufferer either gaining weight from food cravings, or fluid retention, or losing weight because of lack of appetite and anxiety over food. The cry is often, 'All pleasure has gone from eating – just what *can* I eat?'

What is happening?

There can be several reasons for these symptoms. Contributing factors in food intolerances include:

- genetic influence
- stressed immune system

- environmental factors
- harmful bacteria, candida overgrowth, parasites in the gut
- drugs
- inflammation in the gut
- damage to gut wall – 'leaky bowel'
- lack of hydrochloric acid or enzymes
- disturbance of pancreatic function
- low levels of butyric acid made in the gut.

The main one is that a 'leaky bowel' is allowing foreign substances to enter the bloodstream. It can also start in the stomach. Food is meant to reach the bowel in an acceptable state for it to cope with. If there is too much or too little hydrochloric acid in the stomach, or a lack of the enzymes that break down what you eat then this cannot happen.

All stomach problems must be reported to your doctor.

Overproduction of stomach acid

Heartburn or 'acid stomach' is an indication that you are producing too much hydrochloric acid, perhaps because of stress or a diet too high in acidic foods (see *Food Combining for Health* in Further reading). If you have a burning pain in your stomach which is relieved by eating, or if you regurgitate acid, you are probably producing too much acid. Relieving these symptoms with antacids is fine as an immediate measure but only in the short term. If you are tense, the acid–alkaline balance in your stomach can be disturbed. This can be made worse by skipping or rushing meals, and by not eating enough alkaline-forming foods. Water is a good and simple antacid. Drink plenty between meals.

Medical help with 'acid stomach' problems

You might be prescribed a simple antacid or a drug in the cimetidine group such as Tagamet. These drugs are undeniably effective but it is unwise to stay on them for long periods. Unfortunately it is common for repeat prescriptions for this medication to be issued for years.

The drugs can have negative effects on the bowel and the stomach. While they are taken the bowel can be affected by having to deal with food that is only partially digested. Colic, constipation or diarrhoea can result. This clears up when the course of treatment is finished. After withdrawal of the drug the stomach often reacts with rebound overproduction of gastric acid and this can result in an overgrowth of gastric candida.

Drugs such as cimetidine are likely to have an effect on the nervous system. Some people also report experiencing symptoms, after stopping the treatment, of irritability, insomnia, panic attacks and feeling generally very low.

Fungal infections of the skin and further down the gastro-intestinal tract have also been reported with these drugs.

It is a cause for concern that a weaker version of the prescription drug is now available over the counter in the UK. If it helps, use the medication only in the short term (and only after you have had a firm diagnosis from your doctor), but if you feel at all anxious or irritable while taking it you would be well advised to look for a natural approach to the problem of over-acidity, such as changing your diet and lifestyle. If the symptoms persist, see your doctor with a view to further investigations. If your doctor is unwilling to test whether you are producing too much or too little hydrochloric acid, a doctor who practises clinical nutrition will be able to help (see British Society for Nutrition Medicine in Useful addresses – although you might need a referral from your GP).

Too little hydrochloric acid

The body is always striving for balance; therefore it is not surprising that stress can also result in underproduction of hydrochloric acid. It is very confusing because the symptoms can be similar to overproduction of acid and people often compound these symptoms by taking antacids.

Symptoms include excessive burping, a feeling of fullness after even a moderate meal, and bad breath (which comes from food fermenting in the stomach). More severe symptoms include nausea, vomiting, bloating, wind and diarrhoea or constipation. The presence of undigested food in the stool indicates that food is not being digested in the stomach. Proteins (meat, fish, eggs, dairy produce, pulses) are the most difficult foods for the body to digest. Large undigested protein molecules in the intestines can damage the lining and lead to food intolerances, allergies, overgrowth of 'bad' organisms and inflammation which can cause severe diarrhoea.

The production of hydrochloric acid declines with age and even following a good diet can mean that food reaches the bowel in a half-digested state, in which case vital minerals and vitamins may not be absorbed. Eating when you are tired, bolting food or overeating all make hard work for the stomach, and in the case of overeating a small amount of acid has to go a long way.

What can I do?

If your digestion does not improve with antacids or changing your lifestyle and eating habits it could be that you are under-secreting.

- For a few days eat small, frequent, low-protein, high complex carbo-hydrate (whole grains, vegetables, fruit) meals and see if your symptoms improve
- Don't eat when you are tired, and chew your food well.
- Don't drink anything, including water, with meals.
- Wait for at least an hour before you have tea or coffee after a meal.
- If symptoms persist, ask your doctor for referral to a consultant. If this is not possible speak to a nutritionist (see Useful addresses) and ask about betaine hydrochloride, a natural source of hydrochloric acid.

The following conditions often associated with low levels of hydro-chloric acid:

- fatigue
- acne
- IBS
- food intolerances
- disturbances of gut flora
- pernicious anaemia
- asthma
- rheumatoid arthritis
- low immune system.

Lack of enzymes

When food enters the stomach it needs enzymes to help to break it down. If there is a deficiency of these substances then the small intestine has to cope with food that has not passed through the initial stages of digestion. The result is discomfort from wind and bloating. Taking supplements of digestive enzymes or eating a small amount of well-chewed raw vegetables before a cooked meal can help this problem (see *Raw Energy* in Further reading). Pineapple is a good source of digestive enzymes: a piece of well-chewed pineapple or a glass of pineapple juice ten minutes before eating can be helpful. For counselling and information on digestive enzymes see page 89.

The effect of food intolerances on the bowel is discussed in Chapter 7.

Children and food intolerance

Food intolerance in children is becoming increasingly common. Their immune systems cannot cope with modern living: pollution, poor diet and too many antibiotics. They can also be affected by the health of the mother during pregnancy. Children with food intolerances can be pale and listless or pale and hyperactive. Attention deficit disorder can also be a feature. Other symptoms are shown in Figure 3.

Luke

Luke was breastfed until he was five months old and was a contented, cheerful baby. While he was being weaned he became fretful, chesty and had skin rashes. His mother reasoned this was due to teething. By the time he was two years old he was hyperactive and slept fitfully. His mother thought this was 'the terrible twos' and did not seek help until he started nursery school. The teacher said that Luke was aggressive and difficult to control.

When his mother consulted the doctor she was advised to keep Luke on an additive-free diet. This helped, but she still felt that his behaviour was not normal. He could not settle to play with toys or listen to stories

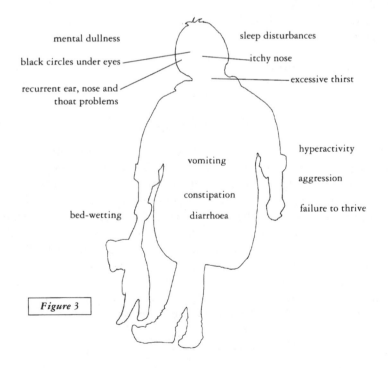

mental dullness

black circles under eyes

recurrent ear, nose and
thoat problems

sleep disturbances

itchy nose

excessive thirst

hyperactivity

aggression

failure to thrive

vomiting

constipation

diarrhoea

bed-wetting

Figure 3

the way her two older children had done, and although she had no doubt that he was intelligent, she noted that at times he was vague, far away and in her words 'difficult to reach'. He was referred to an allergy unit and was found to be intolerant of sugar and anything in the onion family.

One day he came home from having tea at a friend's house and 'appeared in a world of his own'. He climbed on the kitchen table and leapt back and forth from the sink unit and working surfaces. This was something he had never done before. He was aggressive when he was restrained. His mother learned later that he had eaten a vegetable burger containing leeks. There had been similar episodes after birthday parties.

An exclusion diet greatly improved his symptoms; he was calmer, could concentrate and was now quite happy to play alone with Lego or his train set. He progressed well and only lapsed when he strayed from his diet.

In an observational study all cases of a group of children suffering from symptoms of food allergies showed evidence of deficiencies of lactobacillus and bifidobacterias combined with enterobacteriae (harmful bacteria) overgrowth. In another study of infants with diarrhoea the main foods implicated were milk, soy and beef.

Soya products

Many adults cannot tolerate soya products, so it is not surprising that it is high on the list of foods causing problems in children. It seems an unnatural diet for infants when you consider they take up to eight ounces at each feed. Perhaps this, and the fact that they have it every day, is one of the reasons for the development of intolerance: the immune system is constantly bombarded and does not have time to recover. Although high in nutrients, beans can be very indigestible. This could be because they contain both starch and protein (see *Food Combining for Health* in Further reading).

Doctors can prescribe soya milk for babies who are intolerant to cow's milk. While some babies thrive on it, many don't, and both doctor and mother are often slow to suspect the substitute milk because the symptoms do not start immediately. In fact, after discontinuing the cow's milk, there is often improvement for a time. Here is Joseph's story written by his mother. It is a good example of what has just been discussed.

Joseph

When Joseph was six months old I stopped breastfeeding and introduced formula cow's milk into his diet. He developed eczema which got progressively worse. After about eight weeks we decided to remove all cow's milk from his diet. As an alternative my GP recommended specially formulated baby soya milk, available on prescription. The eczema improved considerably and I began using other soya products such as yoghurt and custard. All went well, although I did notice Joseph now drank less milk (about half a pint daily). When he was eleven months old Joseph caught a stomach bug and had sickness and diarrhoea for several days. We gave him water only and he seemed to recover, although his motions remained very loose with a very acrid, sour smell. After a week or so he vomited violently during the night but seemed fine in himself the rest of the time.

This continued for several weeks: violent vomiting during the night once or twice a week. Continued visits to the doctor were unhelpful; I was constantly told that 'babies were like that' or that it was 'just a bug'.

On his first birthday Joseph was very sick again, but this time he was listless, weak and generally poorly for several days. His abdomen seemed swollen and around his anus was sore. I called the doctor but was told not to worry.

After a few days on water only Joseph recovered but by now we were anxious; he seemed to be getting thinner and each illness seemed longer and more severe than the last. This pattern continued for the next couple of months. The bouts of sickness were getting worse and more frequent and Joseph was getting weaker. In between attacks I was giving him as much soya milk as possible in a vain effort to 'build him up'. Finally he was so poorly – this time his abdomen was very swollen and also his feet were swollen – that I demanded hospital admission. He was there for five days and had blood and stool tests. The doctors found nothing and were baffled by Joseph's condition, which by now had improved, although his tummy was still swollen and his rectum remained very red and sore.

I didn't know whether to feel relieved or not. Joseph was discharged and I was told to give him plenty of soya milk and to come back if he became ill again.

By now I was determined to get to the root of the problem and was now convinced of two things: (a) The original stomach bug three months previously had, for some reason, upset Joseph's system so much that he was now unable to tolerate or digest something – but what? Something that had been OK before he got the bug? (b) The solution lay in the elimination of something in his diet, and the sorting out of Joseph's system.

I was continually searching for answers and by now was so stressed myself I didn't know what to do. At this point I decided to seek help from 'alternative' practitioners. I took Joseph to see a homoeopathic doctor and also consulted a nutrition counsellor. Both told me to stop the soya milk and replace it with goat's milk. I diluted the goat's milk at first and built it up to full strength over a week.

Within 24 hours we noticed an incredible difference in Joseph. Soya milk had been the culprit all those months. Joseph seemed almost relieved that we had finally solved the problem. He was altogether happier, his skin cleared, his motions were normal and with the help of homoeopathic remedies and a careful diet (wheat-free and yeast-free), he returned to normal. The counsellor asked if Joseph had ever had oral thrush; he had it three times during the early weeks of his life, and I also have a problem with candida.

Six months after Joseph was ill, he is thriving, his weight is back to normal and he is a really happy child. His eczema has cleared and he now tolerates cow's milk products. When I look back at the whole experience I think that the worst part of it was that not one of the doctors I saw, even at the hospital, suspected intolerance to soya milk. I have since heard of several similar cases. Why is the medical profession unaware of this problem?

IBS due to candida and food intolerances
A case study by Michael Franklin

Susan was a 35 year old from Lancashire who consulted me in the summer of 2005 with extremely bad abdominal pain, bloating and diarrhoea. She gave all three symptoms 10 out of 10 on the scale that we ask people to use in our questionnaires. She also complained of heartburn, indigestion and premenstrual syndrome (PMS). Amazingly, Susan had had to put up with her symptoms for 20 years: they had started when she was 15, and no doctor had ever found an answer. She had been to various GPs and was not able to give any of them more than 1 out of 10 on the GP rating scale we use in our questionnaires.

A very bright person, Susan had read French and German at Oxford, but her IBS symptoms had been so bad that it had spoilt her time as a student and she did not have particularly happy memories of the experience.

Like a lot of people with IBS, Susan had read several times that it is associated with stress. My feeling about this is that stress seldom causes any symptoms or illness but it does, of course, exacerbate them. To blame people's IBS on stress alone is to do a great disservice to thousands of sufferers. There is almost always a sound physiological reason or reasons for their symptoms. The difficulty is to find that reason.

Since I started the IBS and Gut Disorder Centre, after practising as a nutritionist for 12 years, I've always maintained that the four major causes of IBS are:

1   Food intolerances
2   Candida or other yeast infections
3   Unfriendly bacteria
4   Parasites.

Sometimes only one of these is to blame, but in many cases two, three or even all four of them are present in the same person. Unfortunately, people seldom look at more than one. That's analogous to having four nails in your shoe. If you only get rid of one of them, it will still hurt to walk!

The NHS does not look for any of these causes. What usually happens when you go to your GP complaining of constipation, diarrhoea, bloating or abdominal pains is this. Your GP will try and establish whether the symptoms are bad enough to suggest ulcerative colitis, Crohn's disease or advanced stages of cancer. If they do not sound like any of these, he or she will merely tell you that you probably have irritable bowel and that there is not much you can do with it. 'You will have to learn to live with it' is a common remark.

If your GP does suspect any of the three serious illnesses above, you will be referred to a gastroenterologist, who will probably test you with the aid of a camera on the end of a tube which goes down your throat or up from the other end. If it shows nothing, the specialist too will tell you that you have IBS and that there is probably nothing you can do about it.

This is the stage at which most IBS sufferers come to us. Sometimes we can sort out their symptoms just by recommending changes to their diet and treating them for yeast overgrowth, with the aid of natural anti-fungals, the best possible probiotics to restore friendly bacteria, and the right product to heal intestinal permeability, sometimes known as 'leaky gut'. Where the causes are not obvious from the three lengthy questionnaires we use, then we test the patient for food intolerances by means of a blood test (the only scientific way to test for food intolerances) or use the Comprehensive Digestive Stool Analysis to look for any or all of the other major causes: parasites, unfriendly bacteria, candida or yeast overgrowth.

In Susan's case, partly because she did not have too much money to spend and partly because of her answers in the questionnaires, I thought I would try and improve her symptoms just with the aid of probiotics and by changing her diet.

Susan had told me that when she was a child, milk made her retch and feel awful even though she did not remember actually being sick. Hearing this from a patient is very significant because it often suggests either dairy or full-blown lactose intolerance from an early age. Often, in spite of their early bad experiences with milk, the person will have started drinking it again in their teens or, even if they have not gone back to milk, have become a big cheese or yoghurt eater.

This was the case with Susan. In spite of her early childhood experiences, she now ate both cheese and yoghurt every day. I suggested she remove all cow's milk dairy products from her diet along with the two food groups which encourage yeast overgrowth: sugar and yeast. In Susan's case this meant giving up the one or two glasses of red wine she had every evening and avoiding bread, as both of these are major sources of yeast. I also told her to avoid all fruit juice as this is a very concentrated source of fruit sugar and to eat no more than three small portions a week of particular fruits that are low in fructose.

When I next spoke to Susan, only eight weeks later, she reported that the change had been extraordinary. She said, 'My life has been transformed. I'm so much better. I can't believe the difference, my life has really changed!'

Not all cases of IBS are quite so easy to solve. Where we think, on the basis of a patient's questionnaires, that they very possibly have parasites or unfriendly bacteria, then we order a test for these. But where, as in Susan's case, the questionnaires suggest candida and food intolerances, the solution can be very quick to find and the result remarkable.

Michael Franklin
The IBS and Gut Disorder Centre (see Useful addresses)

Food intolerance – the candida connection

Some practitioners believe that overgrowth of candida in the bowel is the major cause of food intolerance. Others believe that it is the other way around: stress and environmental factors cause food intolerance and then candida, the opportunist, takes over when the immune system is too low to fight back. Their answer is to treat the food intolerances first. Omitting the offending foods will make you more comfortable and this is certainly worth doing, but the long-term answer is to stop toxins escaping from a leaky gut (see pages 33 and 40).

Seeking help

Allergy testing in the NHS

During recent years the availability and range of tests for food intolerances in the NHS has increased. Formerly tests were mainly for asthma and hayfever sufferers who were inhaling allergens. Other tests are now available and these include:

The skin prick

This is the standard test to see the reaction to common allergens. A drop of the allergen is placed on the skin, which is then pricked or scratched. If the person is sensitive to the drop there is a swelling of the area known as the weal-and-flare response. This works well for inhaled allergens such as pollens and dust but is unreliable for food intolerances. Sublingual (under the tongue) drops are also used to identify allergens and they are used in diluted concentrations for treatment.

Intradermal injections

These go deeper into the skin than the prick and are more reliable. If the body does not react to the substance, it produces a small weal which soon disappears. In a positive reaction the weal increases in size and becomes white and hard.

Neutralization

This treatment is based on finding a dilution of the offending substance that will 'turn off' the allergic reaction by its influence on the immune system. The reason why this works is unknown, but it seems to have close parallels with the homoeopathic principle of like curing like, that is, the correct dilution of whatever the body considers a poison effecting a cure.

Enzyme-potentiated desensitization

This is more likely to be used by doctors outside the health service who work in clinical nutrition. A mixture of food extracts plus an enzyme are applied in a plastic cup to a scratch on the skin. Desensitization is effected in presumably the same way as described above. One advantage of this method is that it is only needed about once every three months, and less and less often as the immune system recovers. Contact Higher Nature (see Useful addresses) for their latest Immuno Test.

Butyric acid for food intolerance

In a healthy gut adequate amounts of this fatty acid are made by the action of bacteria on dietary fibre (fermentation). It appears in large amounts in breast milk. The lining of the bowel has some of the fastest growing cells in the body and butyrates can supply their energy needs and promote natural healing. Low levels of production could precipitate bowel disease in susceptible persons. Butyric acid has been found to suppress cancer in animal studies and it is thought that it could have a role in the prevention of cancer of the bowel. It should not be used by persons suffering from gastric ulcers or gastritis (inflammation of the stomach). According to one study, some people taking from two to four capsules of butyrates at every meal experienced freedom from many food sensitivities after a period of 7 to 14 days.

Will the doctor be able to help?

The medical evidence for food sensitivities remains controversial because of lack of properly controlled studies; the evidence is mainly anecdotal.

Some people have consulted their doctors for years and have been frustrated with being given endless prescriptions for antacids and preparations for constipation, diarrhoea or colic. Full routine investigations in hospital fail to reveal the cause of their distress, so they just have to live with their symptoms.

Others have been referred by their doctors to the allergy unit of their local hospital and have been able to determine which are their offending foods. Others have found NHS tests for food allergies unreliable (particularly skin pricks) and have had more success following exclusion diets and their own intuition. (A word of caution: Long periods on very restricted diets can lead to vitamin and mineral deficiencies.)

If you can afford to see a doctor who specializes in clinical nutrition you will find that not only will the blood or muscle testing used pinpoint your allergies more accurately, but you are likely to be given much sounder guidance on diet and supplements. If you have to rely on your own efforts, however, do not be too downhearted, because many people have been in the same position and done very well.

The pulse test

A rise in pulse rate can denote food intolerance. Before using the pulse test, avoid the suspected food for at least five days (although some practitioners recommend a month), then take your resting pulse before having a generous helping of the food. Place your palm upwards and press the outer aspect of the wrist with your forefinger, in line with the thumb, and you will feel your pulse.

Count the number of beats in 15 seconds then multiply by four. This will give the number of beats per minute. If it is raised by ten or more beats ten minutes after you have eaten, keep a record of this in a food diary. Take your pulse again after about an hour. Don't rely on memory; keep a record each day of your meals, snacks and drinks and note any symptoms.

Some people don't need to wait ten minutes, or indeed to take their pulse, before their familiar allergic symptoms – heart pumping, headache, wheezing, stuffy nose and so on – descend on them. For some people it takes only two to three minutes. In general the abdominal symptoms take longer to manifest.

Some doctors say that the pulse test is not reliable, reasoning that just because people get anxious and think the food is going to upset them, they experience a rise in pulse rate. This does not explain why people still get reactions when they are not aware of what they are being tested with, as in the 'challenge test' used in hospitals where the patient abstains from certain foods and is then given a solution under the tongue to see the reaction. Neither patient nor doctor knows what is in the bottle.

Ways of helping yourself

How can I find out which food is upsetting me?

The only reliable way is to abstain from foods that you normally eat every day, particularly the ones you feel ill after, and see what happens to your symptoms. The most important thing is to 'listen to your body'. You are most likely to be affected by foods you have eaten most of your life. Dairy and wheat usually head the list. Keep a food diary, taking note of what and when you eat. You may be able to spot a pattern of certain foods being linked with particular symptoms.

Alka-Clear powder

(Available from Higher Nature and New Nutrition) This acid–alkaline balancer not only helps the digestion but benefits the whole body. An over-acid body makes us feel sluggish with headaches, poor digestion, pains and aches and poor concentration. A body in an alkaline state feels calm and energetic. Alka-Clear comes with instructions and urine pH test strips. For best results it should be used with an alkaline diet. A rough guide is three quarters of your plate covered with greens or salads and the rest with protein and complex carbohydrate (see *Food Combining for Health*, Further reading). If you can also keep to eating according to your blood group (see *Eat Right for Your Type*, Further reading) you will feel even better. Don't expect things to happen overnight: keep going and when you are confident that your urine is always alkaline you can stop the powder. The diet should be enough.

Keeping cool

All allergies are worse when you are hot. Try splashing your face with cold water, having a cool shower or bath, or resting with an ice pack on the head or abdomen (don't shudder – this can be surprisingly comforting). Ice packs are available at chemists such as Boots, or the Body Shop. A good alternative is an unopened packet of frozen peas. (The peas can be returned to the freezer but only to be used again as an ice pack – not for consumption!) To prevent 'ice-burn', packs should be wrapped in a thin cloth such as a table napkin or tea-towel.

Food rotation

The principle of this diet is diversification of food. You are most likely to become intolerant of foods you have eaten all your life, and food rotation allows the immune system to recover by not bombarding it with the same allergen every day. Some people react to so many foods that they could not possibly exclude them all because they would become malnourished, so they eat most things, but only once in four days. The body often seems to be able to cope with this and many people do well. It is, of course, tedious, as all these diets are. It involves eating everything to do with the cow – dairy produce and beef – on one day, and everything connected with sheep – lamb, lamb's liver, ewe's milk yoghurt – on the next day, and so on; and also a rotation of different grains, vegetables and fruits every four days. There are many books available that describe food intolerance in detail; see Further reading for some suggestions.

Overweight, candida and food intolerances

Sugar and bread craving (the candida constantly crying out for its favourite food) is probably the main cause of candida sufferers being overweight. Altered hormone levels due to the candida could also be a factor. A genetic inability to cope with grains is another possibility. Many overweight sufferers do not make significant progress until they remove all grains from their diet for at least four weeks. No matter how carefully they have dieted, even on one slice of bread per day, they cannot lose weight. Weight loss is often dramatic when they go grain-free (with the possible exception of brown rice and rice cakes). Fluid retention disappears and bloated abdomens improve even if calorie intake remains the same.

When you eat foods to which you are intolerant, the cells react by protecting themselves with extra fluid. This can dramatically increase weight. The addiction–allergy connection is very close, so you may be craving the very foods that are causing your weight problem.

Some people find it difficult to lose weight because they do not eat enough protein to boost their metabolism and keep their blood-sugar levels stable. This also makes them lethargic and so their problem is compounded by lack of exercise. Vegetarians sometimes fall into this category. Overweight people are often low in essential vitamins and minerals and have a toxic colon problem.

Underweight and candida

If you are underweight, and particularly if your appetite is poor, consult your doctor or a nutritionist before embarking on an anti-candida diet. If your appetite is good and you can eat larger helpings of the allowed foods, and if the weight loss does not continue (you should expect some at first) then you could see how you fare. Underweight people would do well to investigate the desensitization approach (page 42) which only calls for a reduction in sugar and salt.

Water

How many people know that the main cause of daytime fatigue in healthy people is lack of water? Sometimes people think they feel hungry when they are really thirsty. Dehydration can be at the root of many chronic serious diseases, including asthma, kidney and endocrine problems, ulcers, digestive problems and lower back pain. It can also make the memory 'fuzzy'. Every function of the body is monitored by water. Aim for at least eight glasses per day unless your doctor has limited your fluid intake. Many people rarely feel thirsty, but this does not mean you do not need water.

Chemical intolerance

Substances that cause the gut to swell and give rise to other symptoms of intolerance don't always gain access to the body through the mouth; they can be inhaled or absorbed through the skin. Be aware of the chemicals you are spraying on your hair, under your arms, up your nose and on your skin. Use simple non-perfumed toilet preparations and don't buy aerosol cans. Anti-perspirants stop natural detoxification through the skin. Use a simple deodorant; these are widely available. Most essential oils are antiseptic and tea tree (see page 78) is available as a deodorant stick. Some oils come in a carrier oil such as jojoba and can be used as perfume. They smell wonderful and you are much less likely to be affected by them.

Chemicals in the home and garden

It is time also to throw out all the household cleaning agents and get back to simple soaps (non-biological washing powders) and old-fashioned wax furniture polish instead of spray cans. There is a whole range of ecological domestic cleaning products; the washing-up liquid has been particularly helpful for many people. If you cannot find a safe product make sure you immerse the nozzle of your container in water so that you don't inhale the droplets, and also rinse the dishes very carefully. There was research some years ago that confirmed that traces of washing-up liquid can irritate the bowel lining. A tight chest while washing up is also very common in people with chemical allergies.

A simple product called Chemico, a pink paste made from powdered rock which has been manufactured in Britain for about 70 years, is a gentle and safe scouring agent. It cleans everything: sinks, cookers, floors, even windows. You might not find it in the supermarket but a hardware store may be able to obtain it for you.

Avoid garden chemicals as much as possible. Frequent hoeing is safer than using noxious weed-killers and washing-up liquid is quite effective for aphids (unfortunately some plants do not like the ecological products). If you have to paint or use wood preservatives, make sure your working space is well ventilated and that you take frequent breaks.

Travelling

Inhalation of the brake fluid on trains causes swollen eyes, headaches and abdominal symptoms in some chemically allergic people. Travelling by car can also be a problem. Keep the windows closed and if possible fit a car ionizer; they are inexpensive and well worth the effort. Make frequent stops to have a rest from fumes. Chemical inhalants from plastics, adhesives and flooring in shopping areas can also cause symptoms in some people. Printer's ink, tobacco smoke, gas, oil, factory fumes, formaldehyde (air fresheners), chipboard furniture, synthetic carpets – although the fumes from these do decrease with time – are all implicated, in addition to the well-known allergens in nature such as pollens, dust mites and so on.

Parasites

These are far more common than people seem to realize. The common notion is that children might suffer from threadworms from being less aware of food hygiene than adults. This is not the case. A variety of infestations can affect adults and children. These can come from the environment or inadequately cooked foods. The problem is that although the symptoms can be unpleasant they are often confused with other conditions, and even a stool sample does not always reveal the culprit. It can take several samples before an infestation is detected. If you suspect you have parasites you should see your doctor. If this is not helpful, the nutritionists in the Useful addresses section can advise you.

Frozen castor oil capsules for parasites

This method is proving popular and effective. Tigon (see Useful addresses) supply castor oil capsules which you keep in the freezer. This is not like the dreaded weekly dose of castor oil that grandmothers used to give. The castor oil, because it is frozen, is not absorbed in the normal way and therefore does not cause discomfort. The parasites are smothered by the oil and are eliminated. Counselling is available with all Tigon products.

7

A toxic colon

It takes time to clean the colon and to restore the balance of the good and bad bacteria, so be patient. When you have adequate production of enzymes and your dietary intake and internal production of vitamins is correct, your food intolerance should greatly improve or disappear. Colon cleansing is the first step on the road to recovery. It is also vital to cleanse the colon if you have candida problems.

A toxic colon is not only a major factor in the development of food intolerances and chronic vague ill health, it can also cause degenerative disease such as arthritis and cancer. You cannot expect to be well if the main organ responsible for ridding the body of toxic waste is under-functioning.

What is a toxic colon?

If the colon is irritated by diet, stress, drugs, or chemicals, it tries to protect itself by producing more mucous. This binds with the residue from refined foods, such as white flour, and adheres to the wall of the bowel and narrows the lumen. The result is a layer of gluey hardened faeces which can weigh several pounds. Because the bowel is so convoluted this makes an ideal environment for harmful organisms to breed. This layer prevents the production of enzymes and vitamins, and hinders absorption, as has already been mentioned. Do not think that because you have regular bowel movements, or even diarrhoea, that you have escaped this problem. The stool can pass daily through a dirty colon and leave the accumulated residue on the walls behind. There is no need to get panicky about this. The residue of years can be cleaned out. Sometimes the amount of old faeces can be as much as 4.5 kg. This not only causes bloating and all the problems mentioned, but can also be a major cause of lower back pain.

How this toxic layer can affect the body

The effects on the wall of the bowel of this poisonous residue are irritation and inflammation; the general effects include diarrhoea, constipation, fatigue, headaches, dull eyes, poor skin, spots, aching muscles, joint pains and depression. The poisons circulate via the blood through the lymphatic system to all parts of the body.

The lymphatic system

This is a subsystem of the circulatory system. Its main functions are to collect the fluid that surrounds the cells of the body, including plasma protein to the blood, and via this to help maintain fluid balance. It is an important part of the immune system because it produces lymphocytes, which defend the body against disease. It also absorbs fats from the intestines and transports them to the blood. It is a drainage system to rid the body of toxins. It can be seen, then, that a faulty immune system can be the cause of many people being overweight, even when they have a small appetite. Fluid is stored instead of entering the circulatory system in blood vessels in the abdomen and in the shoulder region.

What stops the efficiency of the immune system?

Unlike the circulatory system, the lymphatic system does not have a pump (the heart) to move the fluid around. It relies on movement of the body to do this. The muscles squeeze the fluids into the circulatory system. It is therefore easy to see that a sluggish colon, inadequate exercise and poor water intake render the immune system unable to perform its main function, to protect the body against disease.

A healthy lymphatic system

Healthy lymphatic fluid should serve to nourish cells not fed by blood vessels. The lymphatic fluid also kills off harmful organisms and carries away the refuse. If the body has to pump around excessive toxic waste long term it is not surprising that it sometimes gives up and the disease process takes over. It is understandable that there are more and more people referred to hospitals for irritable bowel syndrome, colitis (inflammation of the colon), Crohn's disease (inflammation of the small intestine), colon cancer and diverticulitis.

When the muscles of the colon wall lose tone, this results in ballooning or the formation of pouches called diverticula, leading to a condition known as diverticulosis. The food trapped in these pockets makes a wonderful breeding ground for bacteria. The result can be diverticulitis, an infection where there is often a fever and acute abdominal pain. This condition needs medical help.

The two diagnoses of diverticula disease and irritable bowel syndrome are often interchangeable. Men are more likely to be told they have diverticula problems, women that they have irritable bowel syndrome. I have covered how to help inflammation of the bowel and the effect of high and low levels of hydrochloric acid in my book *The Irritable Bowel Syndrome and Diverticulosis.*

Cleansing the colon

If the lining of the bowel is inflamed and swollen you could experience of lot of discomfort, and mucous or blood in the stool. Your doctor must always investigate this. Swelling in the lumen of the bowel often produces a flat, ribbon-like stool, which although it is soft can be difficult to pass. Old faeces can cling to the wall of the bowel and cause infection or inflammation. If your bowel is inflamed you will need to gently loosen this material, heal the lining and restore the balance of the gut flora by giving up junk foods and taking supplements. An inflamed bowel should not be attacked by laxatives or taking bran.

The benefits of colon cleansing are manifold, not only in terms of health but also with regard to appearance: the skin looks vibrant; cellulite, water retention and blemishes disappear, and the whites of the eyes regain a youthful clearness.

How quickly you want to clean out is your choice. Some people are so tired of being below par they are willing to endure the effects of rapid cleansing. This does not happen to everyone but it is as well to know that you could experience side effects such as migraine, blinding headaches, nausea, or flu-like symptoms such as aches and pains, fever, exhaustion, and nervous symptoms such as anxiety, panic attacks, irritability, weepiness or even quite profound depression. The worst of this should be over in approximately five days.

You might decide to take the process gradually. Changing to a clean diet over a period of several weeks is described in my book on irritable bowel syndrome. If you also want to lose weight, two books on clean eating with a common-sense approach are *The Wright Diet* by Celia Wright and *Fit for Life* by Harvey and Marilyn Diamond. *Cleansing the Colon* by Brian Wright (available from New Nutrition – see Useful addresses) is an excellent booklet which describes how you can achieve a complete colon cleanse by diet, natural supplements and herbs.

If you cannot afford books or supplements, a diet of 50 per cent raw food would be a good start, together with a teaspoonful of linseed (a bag from the health food shop will last months for little cost) or a dose of Isogel (slowly build up to two level teaspoonfuls), an old-fashioned inexpensive bulking agent available from most chemists. You can chew the linseed to release the nutrients. Isogel is easy to swallow if you mix it with yoghurt or any soft food. It is important to build up the dose slowly as large amounts are likely to cause bloat. Start by taking half a teaspoonful and aim for a comfortable stool at least once a day. If you are constipated take it with a large glass of water. If you have diarrhoea take with just enough to get it down. It swells to a jelly inside and absorbs excess water to make the stool firmer.

Water

Water is essential to clean anything. Aim for two litres per day while you are cleansing the colon unless this conflicts with advice from your doctor. At least a half a pint, preferably hot, before breakfast gets the day off to a good start. Some people say that they can't do that because they retain fluid, but some practitioners believe that the body responds with fluid retention when it does not get enough fluid; it tries to hang on to its ration.

Gentle cleansers

Psyllium husks or powder (available from health food stores or pharmacies) and slippery elm bark (a brown powder available from some health food stores and all nutritionists), taken with plenty of water, are gentle cleansers.

When you start the psyllium you might find it gives you more wind, so start with half a teaspoonful and then graduate to the suggested dosage on the pack, or follow the advice of your nutritionist. This supplement works well but you have to be patient. It could be several days before you are easily passing a soft but formed bulky stool. If your stool is very loose take this supplement with as little water as possible.

You should not have any troubles with the slippery elm. It has a soothing effect on the whole of the digestive system and incidentally is also beneficial for the heart. One teaspoonful three times daily can be taken until symptoms improve.

Colonic irrigation

This simple treatment is a great 'kick start' to getting rid of old faeces and candida. It is unfortunate that it has had a bad press because of people abusing it, thinking it will make them lose weight quickly. People associate this procedure with enemas. There is no comparison. It is not at all uncomfortable; in fact, some people fall asleep during the treatment. It does not involve the retention of water. It is really just like an internal bath. The water reaches much further than in an enema.

You lie on your side in a relaxed position and a speculum is gently inserted into the rectum. Warm sterile water enters by one tube and the old faeces leave by another. The candida may also be seen in the exit tube. It has the appearance of white/grey cotton wool.

How long does it take to clean the colon?

It is unlikely that you will have a pristine inside within a couple of weeks; it could take months. You will know when things are happening: your skin and eyes will look clearer, your digestion will improve, you will have more energy and niggling aches and pains which have been around for years will disappear. You could feel mentally better, too, less jumpy and clearer headed.

Cleansing the bowel and healing with supplements (see below) need not go on for ever. When your symptoms improve you can gradually phase them out and use intermittently when you feel you need it. In addition to the above you will need to avoid stress, keep to a healthy diet, drink plenty of water, and take daily exercise (particularly walking) as much as possible. If you are elderly and cannot move about much, abdominal breathing and simple stretching exercise sitting in a chair will help.

Healing supplements

Magnesium

Candida and ME sufferers are often found to be short of magnesium. Magnesium aspartate is a gentle but effective laxative.

L-glutamine

It is only in the last ten years that it has been found that glutamine is:

- The primary nutrient for the digestive lining.
- The primary fuel for the immune system.
- Vital for the metabolism of muscle.
- Vital for wound healing and tissue repair.
- 'The body's most common amino acid' (Dr Douglas Wilmore, Harvard Medical School).

L-glutamine is an amino acid used by nature to build proteins in the body. One of 20, it was formerly considered non-essential as it was thought that it could be manufactured from other amino acids.

Glutamine in the diet comes from meat, fish and eggs but cooking easily destroys it. There is barely enough glutamine in the diet if we are healthy. Extra glutamine may be needed during times of stress or after illness, infections or surgery.

Glutamine is the most popular anti-ulcer drug in Asia and its success in treating IBS and inflammatory bowel disease is remarkable. The range of illnesses (including mental illness) where L-glutamine is proving to be invaluable is too wide to be discussed here. If you would like more information on this contact Higher Nature (see Useful addresses). This supplement is available through nutritional suppliers in powder or capsule form. It is easier to take adequate doses in the powder form. It is white, tasteless and is taken stirred into water.

Glucosamine (N-Acetyl-Glucosamine or NAG)

This is another very exciting supplement. Clinical studies are showing its value in a wide variety of conditions (for more information contact Higher Nature). Glucosamine is an amino sugar normally formed in the human body from glucose. It works well on its own or with L-glutamine for many digestive problems including IBS, colitis and Crohn's disease. It repairs and protects the lining of the digestive and urinary tract and enables nutrients to be more easily absorbed. It is also essential for healthy joints. Available from nutritionists and health food stores.

Can vitamins help?

A good intake of the B vitamins is essential. Niacin, vitamin B3, is particularly helpful. It has been shown not only to prevent the development of allergies but also to help cramps, and sugar or alcohol craving. It helps detoxification through stimulating the circulation. It has also been found to help nervous symptoms since it closely resembles a group of drugs called the benzodiazepines (Valium, Ativan, etc.).

Niacin can produce a harmless flushing or pricking of the skin which disappears in less than an hour. Nicotinamide is a form of B3 which does not cause flushing. There was a fashion some years ago to give large doses of this vitamin for detoxification, but it was found that patients on sustained medium or high doses sometimes became depressed. This is not surprising, since it has been called 'Nature's Valium'. Valium, or any substance which produces over-sedation, can have this effect.

The B vitamins are synergistic, that is, they depend on each other for absorption (vitamin B3 needs vitamin B6) so it is not recommended that you take any of them in isolation without expert guidance. It is also vital that you choose yeast-free preparations. Some people with bowel problems find that even the purest non-allergenic brands give them problems. If this happens to you, cut down the recommended dose and build up gradually or take them two to three times weekly. More about supplements on page 87.

Aloe vera barbadensis

The juice of this ancient, fleshy plant is the most versatile natural remedy known to modern science. It has 200 constituents including essential vitamins, minerals, proteins, lipids, eight of the ten amino acids necessary for health, and the unique aloe vera polysaccharides.

Aloe vera juice has a number of general benefits. It:

- helps arthritis
- lowers blood pressure and strengthens the heart beat
- lowers cholesterol
- improves liver function
- increases skin and bone healing
- calms and heals the digestive tract
- balances blood sugar levels in diabetes or hypoglycaemia
- helps the immune system.

This list of the helpful properties of aloe vera juice might seem rather long and diverse, but when it is considered that the extract of this plant is detoxifying, anti-inflammatory, anti-bacterial, anti-fungal, and high in vitamins, minerals, amino acids and essential fatty acids, it is not surprising that its applications are so wide.

Aloe vera and IBS

Organic compounds in this juice can all be broken down to form salicylates. These are both analgesic and anti-inflammatory and inhibit the production of inflammatory prostaglandins from arachiodonic acid.

The effect of faulty digestion in the stomach has already been discussed in relation to IBS. Aloe vera can help balance stomach acids, assist in the breaking down of protein and therefore prevent undigested molecules causing problems in the gut (see page 34).

The range of fatty acids produced by the plant includes linoleic, mynistic, caprylic, oleic, palmitic, and steraric acid. Some of these may not only be of value in lowering cholesterol but are also helpful in the production of useful prostaglandins which have anti-inflammatory properties.

Aloe vera has been found to have the anti-inflammatory action of steroid drugs such as indomethacin and prednisolone.

Aloe vera and constipation or diarrhoea

Research has shown aloe vera juice to be an adaptogen, which is a substance capable of reducing diarrhoea, if that is the problem, or in the case of constipation increasing bowel movements.

Will aloe vera juice help abdominal discomfort?

Yes, it will, and there are several reasons why this is so. Improved digestion in the stomach automatically means there is less putrefaction, and therefore, in turn, less gas.

First, food enters the bowel in a more acceptable state, with protein molecules more broken down, which in itself means that less gas will be formed. Second, it helps prevent the overgrowth of bad bacteria and fungus such as *candida albicans*. Too much gas puts pressure on the gut wall, and ballooning or stretching of this wall causes pain. Aloe vera also soothes and heals the inflamed lining of bowel.

More directly, aloe vera also inactivates a potent pain-producing agent and vasodilator (makes blood vessels swell) called bradykinin.

Food intolerance and aloe vera

Again, the juice can be helpful in several ways. It helps prevent large molecules of undigested protein entering the bloodstream. Vitamins and minerals are more readily absorbed and some may be helpful in lowering allergic levels of histamine in the bloodstream. Aloe vera also reduces inflammation caused by food intolerances.

Wind

This is so often the subject of jokes, but it really is not very funny when you 'inflate' after a meal or are wakened in the night by an abdomen so swollen that it is pushing up on your diaphragm and even affecting your breathing.

Most people tend to massage their abdomen to get rid of wind, often without much effect. Try walking around the house firmly massaging the lower back.

Kinesiology

The method here is to identify the offending foods or substances by muscle testing (kinesiology, see page 95) and to stimulate the body's own defence mechanism by giving homoeopathic doses of the allergens. This is known as desensitization. For a practitioner who uses this approach in your area, contact the Institute of Allergy Therapists (see Useful addresses).

8

Chronic fatigue syndrome/Myalgic encephalomyelitis (CFS/ME) and borreliosis

ME is a chronic illness that depresses the immune system. It is thought to be caused by viruses, exposure to certain chemicals (Gulf War Syndrome), pesticides and stress. Another predisposing factor to ME is one that is never mentioned. I have been involved with groups here and abroad for 25 years supporting people coming off tranquillizers and antidepressants, and in the post-withdrawal phase many people are diagnosed as having ME or fibromyalgia. The numbers are too large to ignore. It would make sense because of the effect these drugs have on the immune system.

Because the immune system is so low, other opportunist viruses, bacteria or fungi step in and produce a bewildering, debilitating illness, as you will see in the section on borrelia below. Mainstream medicine is slow to recognize this problem, as I explain.

Those with such symptoms have been classed as malingerers or hypochondriacs for decades, and many have been harshly treated by their medical practitioners. ME was first recorded about 50 years ago, but it is only in the past few years that there has been a sharing of information among sufferers and doctors. It is often mistaken for nervous illness because the symptoms include anxiety, depression and lethargy, and many patients have been labelled hysterics. Scientists have found definite physiological changes in people with ME so there should no longer be any argument; those with ME can be assured that their illness is recognized. Apologies from psychologists, psychiatrists and even physicians are unlikely to be forthcoming but at least those who have been degraded can have their self-esteem restored by having it confirmed that they were not imagining their awful symptoms.

The candida connection

The connection between candida and CFS/ME makes complete sense. The symptom lists are almost identical. Many people who have mistakenly been diagnosed as having ME have completely recovered when the candida symptoms were treated. It also happens the other way around. CFS/ME sufferers frequently have candida problems because of the low state of the immune system, and although they might have other organisms to deal with, getting the candida treated often makes a great deal of improvement.

The borrelia connection

Thankfully, treatment of chronic fatigue is now changing due to the fact that definite physiological changes have been found by dedicated doctors and scientists such as Dr Andrew Wright, Professor Terry Daymond, Dr Sarah Myhill, Jonathan Kerr, Vance Spence, Professor M. Hooper, Professor Anthony Pinching, and many others in the UK. In the USA, Dr William Harvey is among physicians with an interest in this condition, where it is known as CFIDS (Chronic Fatigue Immune Deficiency Syndrome).

Some researchers are finding a link between CFS/ME and borrelia, the bacteria that causes borreliosis, which includes Lyme disease. Lyme disease is caused by a bacteria transmitted by a bite from a wood-tick, which normally lives on deer. Symptoms of the two conditions are often virtually identical, and Dr Wright's work in the UK has also proven that people with CFS/ME often fail to recover because of these kinds of co-infections. The good news is that these co-infections can be treated. In his practice, 95 per cent of people with CFS/ME have tested positive for borrelia.

In the UK health service, tests are unreliable. Often patients are only tested for Lyme disease (borrelia burgdorferi), or for certain European strains of the borrelia organism and even these tests cannot be relied upon. Many people with CFS/ME are so discouraged by the lack of help in the NHS that they do their own research. An email group poll showed that 80 per cent of those with a diagnosis of borreliosis or Lyme disease had a previous diagnosis of CFS/ME.

However, it seems that it might be time for doctors to realize that there are 300 of these organisms worldwide, and infection does not just come from the tick bite responsible for Lyme disease, but also from mosquitoes, fleas, mites and just about anything that bites. It is also passed between humans and in the food chain. It used to puzzle me that not only my clients, but also other members of their family had CFS/ME. Happily, and not before time, things are much more optimistic in this direction.

Many American doctors ignore tests and rely on clinical symptoms for borrelia. Treatment is with long-term antibiotics or botanical extracts such as Samento plus Noni. Dr Wright has written an article entitled 'The terrible trio – infection, inflammation and mitrochondrial dysfunction', which might be of help to your doctor if you have ME and want to be investigated for borrelia. This is available at <www.theoneclickgroup.co.uk> and may be summarized as follows:

Lyme disease is only one part of the much bigger human infection with borrelia species, of which we know very little. There is evidence that borrelia may be much more widespread than previously believed. For example, studies of people in Ireland and Papua New Guinea have shown a surprisingly high prevalence of borreliosis, not related to tick exposure. It seems from this that Dr Wright's exhaustive work confirms what he has said from the beginning: CFS/ME is an infective illness. If you've already had it in the long term take hope – there are answers and more coming all the time.

ME and essential fatty acids

Professor Basant Puri of London's Hammersmith Hospital has proven by MMRI scans that people suffering from ME have enlarged ventricles (spaces) in the brain. This was confirmed by others and the cause was discovered to be a shortage of essential fatty acids (EFAs) and a collection of choline at the base of the brain. Professor Puri used a brand of EFAs which was without docosahexaenoic acid (DHA) (found to be harmful in people with ME) and after three months of these supplements the ventricles returned to normal. All this is described in his ground-breaking book *Chronic Fatigue Syndrome – A Natural Way to Treat M.E.* (see Further reading).

The product, which is called VegEPA <www.vegepa.com>, has many other beneficial effects, including lowering cholesterol, joint health, reduced risk of heart disease, reduced risk of stroke, improved libido, better hair and nails, younger skin (with an actual reversal of the skin ageing process).

How long will it take to see an improvement with VegEPA?

Everybody asks this. Some people see improvements within the first week, but the recommended trial treatment period for ME patients is

12 weeks. The symptoms of ME are so multitudinous that you cannot expect one supplement to cope with all of them within that time; although, I can say, with caution, that a few people have made such progress that they are convinced they will be cured. Be patient and seek advice about symptoms that persist.

What else do I need to do?

Keep your diet as low as possible in linoleic acid, which is found in oils. Professor Puri suggests keeping to virgin olive oil and a small amount of New Zealand butter. New Zealand cows are fed on grass not grains. Most ME patients benefit from being wheat-free and dairy-free. Milk protein and milk sugar (lactose) seem to cause the intolerances, but a little butter may not be a problem. If you want a gluten-free diet, a free booklet is available from NHS Direct, tel.: 0845 4647.

Continue to pace yourself

You may be feeling better, but at this stage remember that you still have ME. Often with the excitement of feeling better, sometimes after years of illness, and being able to achieve even small things, the tendency can be to get 'carried away'. Watch the clock! Rest before pain or fatigue forces you to. Also beware of going back to old habits. When those around you see you on your feet they may expect too much from you. If your partner hints that the kitchen would look lovely with terracotta walls, gently respond by saying that you would like your progress to continue. Likewise don't slip back to running round for the family: let them continue to find their own socks!

Fibromyalgia

Fibromyalgia was not mentioned in Puri's book, but hearing from people who have ME and fibromyalgia, I feel that some have had relief from symptoms that I associate more with fibromyalgia than ME. *The First Year: Fibromyalgia* by Claudia Craig Marek (see Further reading) is well worth reading.

Does VegEPA work for everyone with ME?

While I cannot answer this definitively, I can give some feedback below from several sources, and suggest that you try it.

> *Sue*
> I suddenly realized that I had not used 'artificial tears' for two weeks. I had been using them day and night for three years. My eyes no longer itch and swell. I have only been on them four weeks. Will more things go?

Hari

My insomnia has greatly improved. I did not expect this because of years of disturbed nights. I felt much more tired generally the first week, almost like a drugged feeling and then I could not believe I was sleeping through the night. It's 'swings and roundabouts' with ME. The pain was worse in the mornings and it took me longer to get going but I am doing more and staying up later. This is my sixth week.

Anna

Thank you, thank you for suggesting those capsules. After 15 years of ME how I have longed for even just one thing to change. I reckoned I could not feel much worse so I started on eight a day. I felt a bit sick for a few days (but then, I often do). After four weeks my appetite improved and, bliss, after years of severe constipation and trying everything from my doctor and the chemist, I 'go' straight after breakfast every morning.

Paul

I still feel a bit down, but I am not wanting to cry all the time now and my head pains have diminished a great deal. It's early days, but if the depression continues to improve I will take VegEPA for ever! I feel more like seeing people. I get the same physical feelings each time, almost like a slight cold with sore glands, pressure in my ears, pain all over like toothache (not like ME muscle pain), a huge tummy, nausea, double vision, sore waterworks (but not like cystitis), I feel uncoordinated and have not the energy to think or speak. It comes in cycles. I once had an 'ordinary' depression when I lost a job but it was nothing like this. I first got it when I got the virus that gave me ME. The first sign of it easing is when my tummy starts to go down and then, often in the night my head clears a bit and it's just like somebody putting a light on in my brain. I feel it is possible to go on – until the next time which might be in three days or three weeks. I never know.

It's not all moaning. I have been on the capsules now for nine weeks and I can't say I feel wonderful but my mood is different. I am doing more and for the first time for years I have some hope.

Reading or hearing the experience of others is often reassuring. Keep going!

Do I need to take any other supplements?

It would be surprising if you did not. The best way to do this is to speak with a qualified nutritionist who knows about ME (see page 110). Supplements should be regarded as a medicine. Many people with ME have difficulty taking some supplements, particularly vitamin C because of interstitial cystitis, and B complex because of irritable bowel symptoms. For more on this subject see my book *The Irritable Bowel Syndrome and Diverticulosis*, or see the reference to New Nutrition in Useful addresses, which stocks high quality allergen-free products. If you describe your problem you will be given sound advice. Buy small quantities at first to see if you tolerate them and only introduce one new supplement at a time.

Do I need to see my doctor?

If you have epilepsy or are on medication for any condition it would be wise. It is unlikely that there will be any reason why you cannot take VegEPA. Don't be put off by comments like 'You are wasting your money – just eat fatty fish.' Unless your practitioner can give you a pharmacological reason why you should not take this product, just ignore any negativity.

Essential fatty acid deficiencies in the general population

It could be that in some people there is a genetic predisposition for the body to be unable to utilize from the diet or manufacture in the body EFAs. Apart from the symptoms mentioned in association with ME, if any of the following conditions are in your family or extended family, perhaps you could pass on this information to those affected:

- Hands or feet that become cold or change colour in cold weather. If this is extreme it may be diagnosed as Raynaud's disease. There are drugs for this, but how much better would it be to correct the problem with diet and natural supplements?
- Asthma.
- Allergies, including hay fever and chemical sensitivities.
- Eczema, psoriasis, dry, rough skin, cracked skin around the heels (which can be very painful).
- Needing to pass water more often than would be expected in your age group.
- Hyperactivity and learning disorders in children, including dyslexia.
- Lowered immune function.
- Fatigue.
- Poor wound healing – also associated with zinc deficiency.
- 'Chicken skin' on backs of arms – like permanent 'goose pimples'.
- Hair loss and dandruff.
- Visual problems.

- Tingling in arms and legs.
- High cholesterol.

Diagnosis problems

Working for 25 years in the self-help movement, and judging by the feedback I have had from my books, I never cease to be amazed at the public's intuitive knowledge about their own bodies. 'Doctor, I feel all dried up like desiccated coconut, my eyes, my skin, my hair, my heals crack and bleed and I have had these hard little spots on the backs of my arms since I was a child.' These should be clues for the practitioner, but sadly they are so often missed and the patient leaves the surgery with prescriptions for local applications, or, worse, is seen as a 'time waster' worrying over trivial symptoms. So much illness could be prevented if doctors had more training in nutrition and saw food and supplements as medicine.

In the past, not all ME/CFS/fibromyalgia patients were referred to consultants; but GPs are now much more aware. Things can only improve as more research is done, such as that by the Chronic Fatigue Syndrome Research Foundation which found 15 gene changes in people diagnosed with ME/CFS. The recognition of co-infections in sufferers is another great step forward.

Why am I always tired? Hypothyroidism (thyroid deficiency)

It has been known for over 30 years that blood tests for hypothyroidism are not always reliable. Many people who are a clinical picture of this condition are refused thyroid treatment, even if they have a strong family history. Often they are told their tests are normal or on the lower edge of normal. They suffer the condition for years; it is only when they eventually show abnormal levels that they are given medication. Happily, some informed doctors rely on other ways of diagnosis: the symptom picture, or looking at early morning temperatures taken over a week. Abnormally low temperatures immediately on waking indicate hypothyroidism. In young women this is done away from ovulation time. See Further reading.

Fibromyalgia

This condition often coexists with ME in people who have been on psychotropic drugs. These illnesses can no longer be ignored. They are as real as diabetes or fractures for which people should be taken seriously and have appropriate treatment.

For those who have been treated as 'thick file' patients

Hold up your heads. Many people have had several investigations that have proved normal, and have discovered their problem themselves only through going to an ME group or poring over books or the web. Ask again to see a consultant.

The work of Dr Raymond Perrin for ME

I anticipate that clinics following the Perrin Technique will eventually be established worldwide. This treatment, a manual approach to release toxins, has totally cured many patients since 1989, and has been tested in two clinical trials. Dr Perrin is an osteopath in Manchester who is dedicated to training and monitoring the technique. A DVD showing recovered patients is available (see Useful addresses).

9

Looking for answers

Anti-fungal drugs

Anti-fungal drugs are effective but some are not without their problems.

- **Diflucan (fluconazole)** is increasingly being used for candida. For systemic candidiasis doctors usually give 50 mg a day for two weeks, followed by a single 150 mg dose weekly for several weeks. 150 mg capsules are now on sale over the counter. A single capsule will usually clear thrush. Check with your pharmacist for possible interactions if you are taking other drugs. Also ask about other contraindications. Note: People often consult nutritionists for natural anti-fungal substances after being treated with Diflucan, not only because of toxic reactions but also because they experience a very rapid return of the candida as soon as the drug is discontinued.
- **Amphotericin (Fungilin)** is used for systemic fungal infections and is effective against most fungi and yeasts. It is, however, toxic and side effects are common. They include digestive upsets, headaches and joint pains.
- **Griseofulvin** is well absorbed from the gut and is often used when infections of the skin, scalp and nails have failed to respond to creams and lotions. The side effects are headache, digestive upsets and sensitivity to light.
- **Imidozole group** – clotrimazole, econazole, ketonconzole and miconazole – are active against a wide range of fungi and yeasts. Oral application, except for miconazole which is used for mouth and intestinal infections because of the risk of liver damage, is normally only used in severe resistant infections. The drugs in this group are used widely in pessaries, creams, sprays and powders. Many are available over the counter in pharmacies. They include Canestan (clotrimazole) and Daktarin (miconazole).
- **Nystatin** is an older drug which is not absorbed from the gut This makes it less effective for systemic candidiasis. It is used for intestinal, vaginal and skin infections due to candida. In common with amphotericin it is ineffective against tinea (ringworm).

The side effects can be less than with some of the other anti-fungal drugs, although what is known as the Herxheimer reaction or dieback can occur. As the drug kills the yeast cells they burst and release toxins into the bloodstream. If this is done too rapidly the effect can be similar to flu: raised temperature, headaches, nausea, aches and pains. The problem can be minimized by gradually building up to the recommended dose or by reducing the amount of candida in the bowel by careful dieting for about a month before drug treatment.

The tablets available on the NHS do not dissolve until they reach the large bowel. They would therefore miss infection anywhere else in the digestive tract. This could be helped by crushing them and putting them in water.

With Nystatin powder it is much easier to graduate the dose and it also treats the whole of the digestive tract. If your doctor is willing to prescribe this the supplier could be found through the British Society for Nutritional Medicine (see Useful addresses). He or she may be happier to prescribe this rather than one of the newer non-drug anti-fungals, because Nystatin has been used by the NHS for so long.

Prescribed drugs that favour the growth of candida

Anecdotal evidence suggesting that these drugs can cause candidiasis is overwhelming and there are several references on this subject in medical journals.

- **Antibiotics** encourage candida overgrowth because they are not selective and destroy useful and harmful bacteria simultaneously.
- **The pill.** Disturbances in hormone levels could be one reason why the pill encourages candida. Another could be that in women who take the pill the prevalence of abnormal glucose (sugar) tolerance is increased from approximately 4 to 35 per cent. If the blood glucose levels are raised (hyperglycaemia) there is more food for the candida. This also occurs in diabetes.
- **Corticosteroids** cause hormone levels to be disturbed, and have a much greater influence than other groups of drugs upon glucose tolerance. Drugs like Prednisolone, steroid asthma inhalers and even creams in large doses can have this effect.

  Other drugs that cause raised glucose levels include diuretics, beta blockers, Epanutin3, cimetidine, ranitidine (for gastric ulcers). These drugs are extremely useful for the treatment of gastric ulceration and have saved countless people from surgery.

Unfortunately because they are considered safe they are overused in general practice. They are often prescribed at the slightest sign of gastric disturbance (without a thought to the patient's eating habits or lifestyle) and repeat prescriptions are routinely issued without any reassessment of the patient's condition.

- **Laxatives.** Overuse of strong laxatives prevents the absorption of some essential nutrients and alters the natural bowel flora.

Tranquillizers and irritable bowel syndrome/chronic candidiasis

To my knowledge there have been no medical reports of adverse effects on the gastrointestinal system from medium- or long-term use of tranquillizers, but the mass of anecdotal evidence reporting gastrointestinal problems from tranquillizer groups throughout the world cannot be ignored. No doubt in time there will be scientific research to confirm such findings.

What tranquillizers and sleeping pills do to the gut is unclear but there is no doubt that a very high percentage of users develop irritable bowel syndrome and systemic candidiasis, or some manifestation of fungal infections, during either therapy or withdrawal. Symptoms can persist for years after complete withdrawal of the drugs. More gastrointestinal problems were reported in people taking lorazepam (Ativan) than the other drugs in the group such as diazepam (Valium). It is known that these drugs block the absorption of zinc so it is possible that they hinder the absorption of other vital nutrients and thus allow the body to become depleted; candida thrives in these circumstances. It could be that the benzodiazepines, in common with the drugs mentioned earlier, raise blood glucose levels, thus providing more food for the candida; measurements of blood glucose levels in (non-diabetic) users found that the levels were abnormally high after medication had been taken and dropped below normal when the next dose was due. Cimetidine lowers gastric acid secretion and therefore produces an ideal environment for candida growth.

Some tranquillizer users had also been on long-term cimetidine therapy for symptoms of gastritis caused by withdrawal, but this was only a proportion of those who presented with candidiasis.

Garlic – nature's wonder cure

Garlic is an extremely potent fungicide. Its use in the treatment of candida and many other health problems is highly recommended, except of course for those who cannot tolerate it – its high sulphur content is probably the reason why some people have problems with it. If you know you cannot tolerate anything in the onion family then garlic treatment is not for you. If it merely gives you wind and you have no other signs of intolerance, such as palpitations, headaches or muscle pains, just be patient and your digestive system will get used to it.

During the nineteenth century the medical profession largely turned from the use of natural remedies prepared from plants, minerals and animals, to the use of synthetic drugs. Garlic was known from ancient times for its ability to cure a wide range of ailments: fevers, chest infections, infected wounds, parasitic infection and venomous bites. It was also used for kidney problems and stomach ulcers. The Roman historian Pliny the Elder observed Greek doctors using garlic and recorded:

> It is good for increasing the flow of urine. The best time to eat it is when one is about to drink too much, or when one is drunk. Garlic boiled or roasted is a diuretic, and relaxes the stomach. Garlic causes flatulence, because it stops flatulence.

The last statement may be a reference to what we now know as the homoeopathic principle of like curing like; or it may be that eating foods that cause gas often has the effect of increasing the pressure in the bowel, which in effect carries all before it and allows the trapped wind to be expelled.

Modern research confirms that the historical applications of garlic would have been effective, and also that it is powerful medicine for much that ails our technologically advanced, polluted, toxic, drug-oriented, twenty-first-century world. It has been found to be antibacterial, anti-fungal, anti-tumour, and to be of great benefit to the circulatory system. It also lowers cholesterol levels. Since it is such a powerful cleanser, it detoxifies, eliminating drug residues and environmental pollutants. Chronic cystitis sufferers have found that regular use completely clears their symptoms and obviates the need for antibiotics. Some people find that it lifts depression and gives energy. One woman said, 'I feel as though I'm on wheels.' This may be because in addition to cleansing the body, it is a useful source of trace minerals such as copper, iron, selenium and zinc.

Garlic is effective in a wide range of bacterial, fungal and parasitic infections. Even the fumes from freshly pressed garlic can kill fungus grown on a Petri dish in the laboratory. In the gut, unlike antibiotics, it kills off the harmful organisms, protects against the toxins produced, and encourages the growth of helpful organisms. In addition it aids digestion. Dr Susan Minney writes:

If the active antibacterial compounds within the garlic powder were isolated then, weight for weight, their potency would be very similar to most antibiotics.

Garlic has distinct advantages over antibiotics in that its side effects are very minimal or absent and also that bacteria have not shown any tendency to become resistant to dried garlic.

In summary, the use of dried garlic should be seriously considered in the treatment, or part treatment, of sub-acute, non-life-threatening or chronic bacterial infections, e.g. sore throats, bronchitis, cystitis, skin infections, boils, gastroenteritis and diarrhoea. It is probable that the use of garlic in life-threatening, acute bacterial diseases will always be secondary to antibiotics.

Fresh garlic

This is an inexpensive, safe way to treat candida overgrowth. Its drawbacks are the antisocial effects and for some people the taste. If you (or your family) find these too much to bear you can use one of the deodorized commercial preparations but note that the pills must contain the active ingredient allicin to be an effective fungicide. Most garlic capsules have lost this during manufacture.

Crush one clove (a segment of the bulb) and take immediately either mixed with yoghurt, milk, mashed vegetables or in olive oil drizzled over salad. Wash down with plenty of water. You may feel a burning sensation or slightly sick for a minute but this soon passes and is replaced by a feeling of warmth and, for some, well-being. Do this three times daily with or after food. The fact that the garlic odour can even be noticed on the skin confirms that, in common with one of the television commercials for a certain lager, it reaches parts many other fungicides cannot reach. Incidentally this makes it a good insect repellent.

Garlic can also be usefully absorbed through the skin; garlic rubbed on a baby's feet can be noticed on its breath. Miners used to put fresh cloves of garlic in their clogs to keep them free from chest infections. For a fascinating history of the use of garlic and how to prepare inhalations, and external remedies see *Garlic: Nature's Original Remedy*, by John Blackwood and Stephen Fulder (see Further reading).

Health food stores stock garlic products but the quality can be variable. Garlicin, from BioCare, a biotechnology company with a team active in the field of garlic research and the capability to produce a consistently high-quality products, can be ordered by post (see Useful addresses).

The garlic experience

Here are the stories of two people who ignored the pleas of their families and completely cured their symptoms by using fresh garlic.

Julia

Julia was, in her words, 'in a state'. She had recurrent thrush and cystitis, and her face was bloated and covered in blemishes. Every few weeks she developed a cold, mouth ulcers or cold sores on her mouth or inside her nose. Her other problems were weight gain and a persistent rash on her upper arms and chest. She had a history of taking street drugs and abusing alcohol but had been drug-free for two years and only drank at the weekends. Her diet was yeast- and sugar-laden and her only exercise was walking to college some 15 minutes from her home.

Having found some answers and a plan of action, she felt less depressed, and after a week on fresh garlic, a clean diet and taking more exercise she could already see physical improvements; her bladder problems had gone. Three weeks later she was greatly improved; she had lost five pounds in weight, and the spots on her face had cleared. The itching and burning in the vulva had gone and the discharge was much less. She had been using a douche of two crushed garlic cloves to a pint of warm water. Straining the garlic water before use avoided 'bits'. She continued taking garlic, with occasional lapses, for six weeks and kept to her new eating plan. The rash on her arms and chest improved over the months but did not finally clear until she used Canestan cream. Within three months she felt 'a totally new person'. For Julia it was also an exercise in self-assertion, as she had to disregard the complaints of the family. Since she had often been told she 'never finished anything', her self esteem was boosted by the fact that she had completed her treatment.

Julia's story illustrates how discouraging it is to work hard to be drug-free, and then to be confronted by a new set of problems. There is very little information around on what can happen in the body after withdrawal from street drugs or when some medications are reduced or withdrawn.

John

John had suffered from a bowel infection while travelling in India a year earlier. Hospital tests had all been negative. He complained of feeling lethargic, bloated, of loss of appetite and more recently of a rash around his genitals. He was vegetarian and did not like sweet foods so his diet needed little adjusting. He was in the middle of a three-week colon cleanse prescribed by a herbalist. This had given him diarrhoea, but he knew that was all to the good. He took three cloves of raw garlic daily and in addition often had it cooked in his meals. He increased the protein in his diet and took yeast-free nutritional supplements. Within a month he felt stronger and while he was still bloated he was not so uncomfortable and his appetite had improved. His energy returned and the fungal rash cleared with sea bathing and sunshine.

John's experience highlights the fact that when you are using garlic, the precise nature of the infection does not really matter, because it deals with pathogenic bacteria, fungi or parasites. Whether it was a candida overgrowth due to a stressed immune system or whether it was a parasite he had picked up on his travels, garlic effected his cure.

Other non-drug anti-fungal substances

Caprylic acid

This fatty acid is a component of certain food fats that have been included in our diet for centuries. It works selectively to inhibit the growth of yeasts, leaving lactobacillus unharmed. It is found in large quantities in breast milk. Commercial preparations are made from coconut oil and are available from most health food stores. Mycropryl, from BioCare, is reliable and is also available in junior strength. It is very effective and side effects are rare, but it should not be used by people with gastritis, gastric ulceration or intestinal ulceration.

Citricidal

This is an excellent product, available from New Nutrition. It is anti-fungal, antibacterial, anti-parasitic, and also has some antiviral activity. Popular for some years, it comes with a leaflet describing its great variety of uses, including disinfecting food, utensils and laundry. It is not only for fungus. Many people have found that one dose can clear diarrhoea or gargling quickly cures a sore throat. It is of great value to take when you are travelling abroad. Counselling is available.

Exciting newer botanical antibacterials, anti-fungals and antivirals

There is not space to do these extremely helpful substances, including olive leaf extract and oregano oil, justice here, but there are some remarkable testimonies on the web and reports from candida and ME groups.

Botanical extracts cope with a very wide range of organisms without the toxic side effects of drugs. These are available from Tigon and although they come with information leaflets, it is worth buying the low-priced books that explain the science behind the claims. Counselling is available.

The products are quite powerful, and the same care to avoid experiencing symptoms from 'die off' has to be taken as with anti-fungal drugs. 'Die off' is when the toxins from the dead yeast cells flood the system. This can make you feel as though you have a severe bout of influenza. If you kill off the candida slowly you can minimize this effect.

In the case of oregano oil, although many people have found this very helpful, some who suffer from irritable bladder have found it too strong even in the lowest dose.

Mary

I have ME/borrelia. I had to take Samento and Noni for the borrelia long term. Within 48 hours of starting them I had terrible thrush. I always get this with antibiotics so I felt they must be working. Anti-fungal drugs, creams and pessaries did little to help, but one olive leaf capsule per day kept it well under control. I was so pleased I had read about it.

For more information on botanical extracts see Useful addresses.

Herbs

Berberine is present in a number of medicinal plants including goldenseal, oregan grape and barberry. These plants have been used in the treatment of diarrhoea in India and in traditional Chinese medicine for 3,000 years. *Artemisia annua*, another traditional Chinese herb, is used for intestinal parasites. A formula containing all the above substances is marketed under the name Eradicin Forte. Tricycline is a similar product (available from BioCare). These products are very effective and can be used with other products such as caprylic acid or other anti-fungals. They should not be used during pregnancy. This is the only contraindication issued by the manufacturers.

The science of probiotics

This is the use of live bacterial supplements to kill off harmful bacteria in the gut and restore balance in the gut flora. The benefits of lactobacillus acidophilus have been known for over a hundred years and have become a routine part of nutritional and preventative medicine.

Nutritionists believe that many degenerative diseases begin with distur-bances in the gut bacteria. After cleansing, the colon needs to be recolonized with helpful bacteria. Health food shops stock bacterial supplements but these cannot always be relied upon to contain live bacteria. It is better to order from a company (BioCare, New Nutrition) whose products have this guarantee. If you are milk intolerant you will need to look for a milk-free strain.

Live yoghurt will provide you with some helpful organisms but it is unlikely that this will be enough to recolonize the gut if you have a candida problem. The newer 'live' yoghurt drinks can be helpful. New Nutrition have a product especially made for use with antibiotics.

ThreeLac

This is very popular in the USA. Anti-fungal treatments do not need to be taken with this product. It is a formulation that includes three strains of live lactic acid bacteria: spore forming lactic acid bacteria (*bacillus coagulans*), spore forming bacteria (*bacillus subtilis*) and lactic acid bacteria (Group D [non-toxic] *enterococcus faecalis*). The bacteria gets into the intestines alive and unharmed.

Other ingredients include lemon juice powder (for flavouring), refined yeast powder (a small amount, which simply feeds the ThreeLac; it does not affect yeast-sensitive individuals), and fibre (FOS, which feeds the bacteria). It also helps to maintain the body's pH and does not interfere with other medication, although it would be wise to take it away from the time when you take antibiotics. Available from nutri-tionists in the UK and the USA.

Homoeopathy and candida
by Elizabeth Edmundson

Hippocrates stated that he would rather know what sort of person had a disease than what sort of disease a person had. He went on to say:

> A physician who is an honour to his profession is one who has due regard to the seasons of the year and the diseases they produce; to the states of the wind peculiar to each country and the quality of its waters; who looks carefully at the locality of towns and of surrounding country, whether they are low or high, hot or cold, wet or dry; who moreover takes note of the diet and regimen of the inhabitants, and, in a word, of all the causes that may produce disorder in the animal economy.

First, it is necessary to discuss the principles of homoeopathy in order to understand how we arrive at the appropriate remedy. It is this remedy that strengthens the fighting ability of the body towards disease, in this case candidiasis.

Conventional medicine treats the symptoms that the person presents. On the other hand, the homoeopath treats the whole person. For instance, take an arbitrary figure of five patients with acne. The orthodox practitioner will treat all of them similarly, whereas the homoeopath, because he or she is treating the person as opposed to the symptoms, may end up prescribing different remedies for each of them. Although they all have acne, the disease has manifested through different medical backgrounds with varying causes. The homoeopath takes a detailed history, looking at the uniqueness of the individual. The purpose of this close scrutiny is to elicit enough information to paint a picture, thus enabling a remedy selection appropriate to the totality of the person's symptoms. The potency of the remedy is then selected, which ideally matches the dynamic plane of the disease at that time. When the remedy and potency have been chosen, this is called the *similimum*, and when the patient picture matches the remedy picture progress is almost guaranteed.

Principles

- **The foundation of homoeopathy** is *similia similibus curantur*: 'like shall be cured by like' or 'that which makes sick shall heal'. Samuel Hahnemann, the founder of homoeopathy, states that the matching remedy for a disease is a substance which in a healthy person produces the same symptoms as displayed in the sick person.
- **The single remedy.** All the symptoms are arranged in order of importance, and the remedy is given. The principle of the single remedy treating the whole person is in sharp contrast to the allopathic system where often multiple drugs are prescribed at one time.
- **The minimum dose.** Very minute doses of the selected remedy are administered. Hahnemann discovered that by reducing dosages unwanted aggravations were reduced and yet the remedies were still effective. He went on to develop a system of diluting remedies to a point where not a single molecule of the original substance is present, only its energy pattern. He called this process of repeated dilution along with succussion or shaking, potentization. (In the old days succussion took place on the family Bible, whereas nowadays machines are used.) Apparently it is in the succussion that curative

properties are released and believed to work on the deeper subtler spheres of the human being, so the higher the potency the smaller the amount of the medicinal substance present in solution.

- **Provings.** Substances used are from animal, vegetable and mineral sources. Their potential healing properties are tested on healthy persons where there is no risk of results being tainted by a disease picture. Hahnemann in fact dosed himself with Peruvian bark and eventually 'tipped over' into full-blown symptoms of malaria. When he stopped taking the medication he became well again. Today this substance is used homoeopathically in the treatment of malaria.

How does homoeopathy work?

At the centre of homoeopathy is the concept of the Vital Force. World philosophies recognize this unseen energy – prana, ch'i, bioenergy. When the body manifests symptoms they are seen as the visible expression of the disturbed Vital Force. Orthodox medicine sees symptoms as evidence of a morbid process that must be eradicated or suppressed, and it puts great store by the study of pathological change, chemical disturbances, bacteria and viruses, which leads to treatments directed against them. Homoeopathy, on the other hand, views illness as a dynamic disturbance of the Vital Force and it is that which must be restored to full functional harmony.

Symptoms are simply the result of a disease and not its cause. In health the Vital Force keeps the 'clocks wound', whereas in sickness the clocks 'wind down' because the immunity is weakened and symptoms develop. When the remedy is given, this stimulates the immune system into action again.

How will this help our patient with candidiasis?

In my experience this problem is best tackled using dietary means, with suitable supplements (recommended is the Cantrol Pack available from Health Plus Ltd – see Useful addresses) taken concomitantly with the selected homoeopathic remedy. It is important to stress that although the candidiasis can be fairly easily treated, underlying causes must be addressed: for example, repeated antibiotics for recurring sore throats – homoeopathy will reduce that predisposition.

Case 1: 32-year-old female, L. A.

Complained of:

- halitosis (teeth checked – musty odour)
- bloating and belching after meals

- prone to sore throats – frequent antibiotics
- craves sweets and chocolates
- allergies to lanolin and topical alcohol
- strong light induces migraine
- no energy or stamina
- poor memory
- muscle weakness
- poor, unrefreshing sleep.

She had been on the pill for nine years.

Progress: Marked improvement after one month. Required further treatment for three months. Homoeopathic remedies effectively strengthened her immune system. She married in six months and discontinued the pill. Prolonged exposure to the pill and frequent courses of antibiotics I felt were the culprits.

Case 2: 23-year-old female, J. H.

Complained of:

- severe depression for two years – prescribed antidepressants by psychiatrist
- feels alone, forsaken, suicidal, weepy, worse in morning
- 'as if seeing things out of focus'
- 'as if out of touch with reality'
- 'no middle moods'
- 'fears something will happen'
- easily stressed
- poor sleep
- recurrent tonsillitis, treated with antibiotics – always 'low' afterwards
- profound energy lack – wondered if had ME, severe PMS.

Progress: Drugs slowly reduced under supervision. After one month a dramatic improvement mentally. It took nine months for her to be symptom-free, and now this patient is in control of her life.

Homoeopathy is a powerful and necessary facet of candida treatment, because it treats the cause – why the patient becomes susceptible initially.

Elizabeth Edmundson is a trained nurse and midwife and a registered homoeopathic practitioner. She has had an interest in candida problems for many years and uses a combination of homoeopathy, supplements and diet.

Essential oils

It must be said before any discussion of the benefits of essential oils that while many of them can safely be included in self-help care, they are powerful substances and some are toxic. It is therefore important to follow the instructions of a qualified aromatherapist or use only the oils recommended in aromatherapy books. There are some excellent ones available which give clear instructions on choosing and mixing oils for everyday problems such as tension, headaches, indigestion, lethargy, anxiety, depression and so on. Essential oils can also be of great value in home beauty treatments. Please note that beauty therapists are trained in the use the oils only to promote relaxation and for skin care; they are not able to apply them for specific medicinal effects (i.e. aromatherapy).

The medicinal value of distilled oil from plants, fruit, wood and resins has been known for thousands of years. During the past 40 years there has been a resurgence of interest in their use and medical research has confirmed that they are not merely pleasant smells that relax or stimulate the body, but that they have great value in alleviating or curing a wide range of physical and emotional conditions. They can be administered through the skin, through inhalation or orally.

When mixed with a base or carrier oil they are absorbed through the fatty tissue of the body during massage. A 20-minute soak in a warm bath containing a few drops of oil allows the same penetration. When inhaled from a tissue, in hot water or from an oil burner, the vapours enter a primitive part of the brain called the limbic system. Tranquillizers also use this part of the brain.

Except where instructions clearly state that oils can be taken orally, for example one drop of peppermint oil in a glass of warm water for the relief of wind, they should not be taken internally unless prescribed by a qualified aromatherapist.

Many of the oils have bactericidal and fungicidal properties; the most important one for candida is tea tree.

Tea tree oil for candida and other problems

For thousands of years the Bundjalung Aborigines of Northern New South Wales have valued the healing properties of the tree *melaleuca alternifolia*. There are over 300 varieties of the tea tree but only one produces the medicinal oil. Research shows that pure tea tree oil is an extremely complex substance containing at least 18 organic compounds that work together in synergy to produce maximum healing benefit.

The first European to collect samples of the leaves was Joseph Banks in 1770. About the same time Captain Cook's sailors made a 'spicy and refreshing tea' from the leaves to replace the tea they had brought from England – hence the name.

In 1922 an Australian chemist conducted experiments and announced his results to the Royal Society of New South Wales. He discovered the very high antiseptic power of the oil: 13 times stronger than the carbolic acid that was used at the time (it is now known that it is four times stronger than modern household disinfectants). His findings prompted more research and in January 1930, under the heading of 'A New Australian Germicide', the editor of the *Medical Journal of Australia* reported on the use of the oil in general practice.

> The results obtained in a variety of conditions when first tried were most encouraging, a striking feature being that it dissolved pus and left the surfaces of infected wounds clean, so that its germicidal action became more effective without any apparent damage to the tissues.

In 1930 the *British Medical Journal* stated: 'The oil is a powerful disinfectant, but it is non-poisonous and non-irritant, and has been used successfully in a very wide range of septic conditions.'

Although it was found to be effective in so many conditions, including fungal skin problems, demand outstripped production and synthetic germicides were developed. With the advent of 'miracle drugs' (starting with synthetic penicillin) the value of tea tree was overlooked. In the 1970s, however, there was a renewal of interest in the oil and it is now available in a wide range of products world-wide.

Tea tree oil can effectively treat a great number of ailments, due to its healing and infection fighting properties, including athlete's foot, toenail infection, acne and dermatitis, mouth ulcers and cold sores, and a number of other complaints associated with candida and fungal infections. Its value in treating thrush and cystitis is described on page 15. You will find tea tree oil in most stockists of essential oils. Thursday Plantation (see under Optima Health and Nutrition in Useful addresses) is a reliable brand. They also produce a range of skin and hair care products and offer an excellent leaflet detailing the uses of tea tree oil.

10
Diet

It is impossible to set out a candida diet that would suit everyone. There are so many approaches to diet for the control of candidiasis that if you read a several different books on the subject you could end up being totally confused. Some practitioners insist on very strict regimes; others say that what you eat isn't important if you are on anti-candida medication, you can eat what you like (this would seem to be going too far, progress would be slow). Others say keep to a diet but don't worry if you have an odd lapse, just take an extra dose of your anti-fungal substance. Before you read on and get discouraged by the idea of a restricted diet there are other ways (see page 42 on desensitization), although remember that you are unlikely to recover from any condition if you abuse your body with junk foods, excessive alcohol and so on.

The right diet for you

Your personal choice will obviously be determined by likes and dislikes, the severity of your symptoms and how desperate you are for them to disappear, food intolerances, and how much stress is involved for you in rigid dieting. This chapter suggests both a moderate approach (Diet 1) and a strict anti-candida diet (Diet 2). You might choose to follow Diet 2 for the first three weeks, to get your treatment off to a good start. Very restricted diets should be avoided for long periods, however, not only because of the danger of your intake being nutritionally narrow but also because eating should be a pleasure and not a continual worry. Remember, stress encourages fungal growth.

Diet as a medicine, not a punishment

It's best to think of approaching the candida diet not as a life sentence to an unpleasant diet, but as a temporary change to improve your health. While you are on the diet, after the first month you can have the odd lapse, and then as your symptoms disappear, you can look forward to a more normal, but still healthy, way of eating. A diet laden with refined sugars and fats is dangerous for everyone, with or without candida, so it is envisaged that you will never go back to that; it is unlikely that you would want to after you have experienced the difference in your well-being while eating healthily. Be kind to yourself, particularly if you have been eating carbohydrates or drinking excessively for comfort. You might feel anxiety or grief at having to give up your 'security blanket'. So often the cry is 'But I cannot live without bread' – you can, and you will, if it is necessary and if you really want to get better.

The following are guidelines to starve the candida:

- Absolutely fresh foods.
- No refined carbohydrates.
- Restrict unrefined carbohydrates.
- Aim for a diet as low as possible in yeast.
- Avoid or cut down on foods which contain antibiotics or steroids.

Overripe fruit, limp vegetables and bread that has been around for a few days all harbour mould spores. If possible, shop for smaller quantities from stores that have a rapid turnover of produce. Take extra care over storage of food; wash out the bread bin regularly or store bread in fridge. If you are using only very small quantities, slice a loaf as soon as you buy it and freeze it. You can take your ration out daily. It defrosts quickly or can be toasted from frozen.

Diet 1: moderate approach

Avoid or cut down on:

- sugar, white or brown
- treacle, golden syrup
- molasses, sucrose, glucose dextrose, marmalade, jam
- white flour and all products made from white flour: cakes, buns, teacakes, biscuits
- all processed grains including some prepared breakfast cereals
- yeasty foods: hard cheese, blue cheese, marmite/vegemite, brewer's yeast or any supplements containing yeast, vinegar and all fermented products
- alcohol, fizzy drinks, fruit squashes
- dried fruit
- tinned fruit in syrup.

Eat:

- whole grains: whole grain bread, pasta, brown rice, any other unrefined grains
- puffed wheat, puffed rice, shredded wheat – all sugar-free, also sugar-free muesli or homemade muesli
- meat, poultry, eggs, dairy produce: milk, cream, butter, cottage cheese, soft cheeses, fromage frais, yoghurt – preferably plain or diet
- fish – fresh or tinned
- legumes: lentils, peas, beans, chickpeas
- nuts and seeds
- spices
- fresh or dried herbs
- large quantities of vegetables, raw or cooked
- useful thickeners for soups and stews: arrowroot; grated potatoes; additive-free vegetable stock (Marigold bouillon, widely available)
- fresh fruit
- olive oil, any other vegetable oil, margarine or butter
- low-sugar jam
- diet drinks (in moderation)
- fructose (fruit sugar), honey (in moderation)
- dry white wine or spirit with low-sugar mixer or water (in moderation).

Diet 2: strict approach

You could use this for three weeks to get a good start, or before starting anti-fungal drugs/substances. This would minimize the die-off symptoms.

The following foods are banned:

- sugar, white or brown; treacle, golden syrup, molasses, sucrose, glucose dextrose, any product containing sugar
- white flour and all products made from white flour: cakes, buns, teacakes, biscuits
- pasta, white rice
- all prepared breakfast cereals
- cured products: bacon, kippers, smoked salmon
- all fermented products, vinegar, pickles, chutney, sauerkraut, tofu, soy sauce
- alcohol
- tea, coffee, cocoa, Ovaltine, Horlicks
- any malted product

- all dairy produce: milk, cheese, cottage cheese (with the possible exception of live plain yoghurt)
- mushrooms, truffles
- dried fruit
- fresh fruit for first three weeks
- spices, dried herbs
- tinned foods
- artificial sweeteners, diet drinks
- nuts
- citric acid
- cream of tartar.

The following foods are allowed:

- restricted whole grains: up to 80g per day (one small slice of whole grain bread = 30g)
- brown rice, Ryvita, rye bread, rice cakes, oat cakes, whole oats, millet, buckwheat, barley
- wholewheat pasta, wholewheat noodles, buckwheat pasta
- free-range chicken, eggs, turkey, duck, rabbit, lamb, venison, fresh fish, shellfish
- legumes: peas, beans, lentils, chickpeas, etc.
- seeds: sunflower, sesame, linseed, pumpkin
- all vegetables (eat mountains of them), raw or cooked
- sea vegetables
- well-washed, peeled fruit.

Why certain foods are banned

All the foods on the formidable 'banned' list either feed candida, or contain additives to which chronic sufferers could have intolerances. Bloom on the surface of fruit is mould, and nuts and spices often harbour mould. Some nutritionists ban artificial sweeteners because some of them are made from sugar (Nutrasweet and saccharin are not) and they believe that their inclusion in the diet perpetuates a craving for sugar.

Some lifelong tea and coffee drinkers can abstain without any problems. Others can have what is known as the 'caffeine storm'. This is when all the caffeine in the body is mobilized and before it is eliminated it can cause severe headaches, nausea and aches and pains. A cup of tea or coffee usually eases the symptoms within half an hour. If this happens to you phase tea and coffee out gradually.

Sugar

You do not need sugar for energy. On the contrary, it can drain away your energy. Sugar is not only empty calories, it is the food of choice for candida and it prevents the absorption of essential minerals and vitamins. It also plays havoc with your blood-sugar levels and disrupts the function of your pancreas, causing a multitude of unpleasant symptoms including panic attacks. The importance of keeping blood-sugar levels stable is explained fully in my book *Coping Successfully with Panic Attacks* (Sheldon Press, 1992).

Sugar in tea or coffee should be stopped immediately. You will get used to it eventually and if it makes you cut down on tea and coffee, so much the better. Try not to turn to regular use of artificial sweeteners; this just prolongs the desire for sweet drinks. Occasional use of sweeteners or a diet soft drink can be regarded as a treat. Withdrawal or sugar craving causes some people to abandon the diet. If you feel in danger of doing this use very small amounts of fructose, fruit sugar (this looks like sugar and is available from pharmacies and health food stores), or honey. These do not disturb the pancreas and are less likely to trigger yeast growth. Look for honey from bees that have not been fed sugar. Organic honey is best but there may be other brands that are less expensive.

Refined carbohydrates (sugar and starches)

All refined grains and products made from refined grains encourage yeast growth. They have also lost many essential nutrients in processing. Diets high in refined starches are the main cause of toxic colon syndrome. The starch combines with mucus in the gut and forms a gluey layer, which collects on the bowel wall. The effects of this are described in Chapter 7. There is little argument about the inclusion of refined carbohydrates in the diet; most nutritionists recommend their avoidance, except perhaps where someone with a wheat intolerance finds white bread, particularly toasted, less of a problem.

Diet drinks

Some people imagine that because diet drinks are sugar-free (although check labels because some sweeteners are sugar-based – Nutrasweet is not) that it is fine to drink as much Diet Coke as you like. Since you are trying to clean chemicals and additives from your system this does not seem a good idea. All soft drinks contain citric acid. This encourages yeast growth and can also make cystitis sufferers very uncomfortable. You could make your own soft drinks from freshly squeezed fruit juice and carbonated water.

Newer sweeteners may contain fewer additives: Splenda is advertised as additive free but it is made from sugar; and any such product will, of course, maintain the desire for sweet food.

Dairy products

There is a division of opinion on dairy products. Some practitioners recommend them particularly for underweight people, and believe lactic acid to be helpful in candida problems; others discourage their use. Dairy products are mucus-forming and it would be well to avoid them if you have chest or catarrhal problems, if you are intolerant to them or if you are on a colon-cleansing programme. Otherwise go by how you feel if you include them.

Eggs

It is a pity that eggs have had such a bad press lately. Egg yolks are rich in essential nutrients and also help to keep the bowel flora healthy. If you are not in a high-risk heart disease group and if eggs are eaten as part of a healthy diet, their cholesterol content is not a problem. A well-cooked egg is a useful addition to the anti-candida diet. Free-range eggs do not contain antibiotics.

Complex or unrefined carbohydrates

Whole grains and products retain all their nutrients and because their fibre content has not been discarded give the stool bulk and stimulate peristalsis (the contractions and movements in the bowel), thereby keeping it clean. Bacteria acting on the cereal fibre prevent fungal growth. Complex carbohydrates are broken down slowly in the body and release a steady flow of glucose into the blood which prevents the 'kangarooing' of blood glucose levels, with its resultant drop in energy and craving for sugary foods.

There is a division of opinion on whether to restrict complex carbo-hydrates. Some practitioners say eat as much as you wish of any whole grain you can tolerate. Others restrict them, saying that they still encourage fungal growth even if they are unrefined.

Will changing my diet affect me?

It could, particularly if you have been accustomed to a high refined carbohydrates menu. You might experience withdrawal symptoms, including sugar craving. Change of diet and/or the addition of supple-ments can also produce lethargy and aches and pains in the first few weeks. Be prepared for this and welcome it: it can be the candida dying off or the effect of other toxins being released from the body.

Diet for an inflamed bowel

This is not strictly an anti-candida measure but can be a help to soothe the digestive tract, clean the colon and give the liver and kidneys a rest before you start anti-candida treatment. It is a diet for people whose digestive symptoms have been fully investigated by their doctor.

Savoury

Simmer for an hour and a half a large pan of any fresh vegetables, root and green (even lettuce), except those in the onion family, plus parsley or any fresh herb of your choosing. Add Marigold bouillon stock powder or vegetable stock cubes.

Use this stock (but do not eat the vegetables) to cook white rice. Cook the rice well. If you can bear it, it is better to use plenty of stock, give the rice a long slow cook and eat it as a thick soup. If this does not appeal, it is fine to cook it less and have it as separate fluffy grains. Sprinkle with a little rock salt or Marigold stock powder if it is too bland for your taste.

Sweet

Cook white rice with a little rock salt. Have this hot or cold with plain yoghurt and a little honey or apple juice.

Supplement

Take one teaspoon of slippery elm bark (not the slippery elm drink with added milk but the pure bark available in whole food shops), in water, three times daily. This is also available in tablet form from health food stores. Isogel, an inexpensive, soothing bulking agent available from chemists, will have a similar effect although some people say it gives them wind.

Drink plenty

Preferably water (bottled if possible), and herb teas; if you get a headache, one or two cups of weak tea or coffee per day maximum.

Don't wait for meal times

Eat either the savoury or sweet rice whenever you feel like it during the day. Do not allow yourself to get hungry. If you are underweight don't continue the diet for any more than two days unless you are managing to eat good quantities. If you are overweight you could continue for seven days – the bathroom scales will please you! You might find it boring but nothing is more boring than the nagging soreness of an inflamed digestive tract.

The value of fresh raw vegetables and fruit

This cannot be overemphasized, not only from a nutritional point of view but also as an aid to digestion, to cleanse your system and for enzyme production. Since these are complex carbohydrates you can eat them freely. Many people who have problems with cooked vegetables can eat them raw without producing symptoms. If you prefer them cooked, eat a small salad before your meal or nibble some vegetables as you prepare them. Remember the keyword is fresh; there is a great deal of difference between the juice from a fresh orange and a glass of orange juice from a carton.

An exciting book on the energizing effects of raw foods, sprouting seeds and how to cleanse with vegetable and fruit juices is *Raw Energy* by Leslie and Susannah Kenton (see Further reading).

Nutritional supplements

People often comment that they are bewildered by the rows of supplements in health food stores. The following is a guide to help you choose ones that help to boost the immune system. However, if information here on the choice and dosage differs from that suggested by your doctor or nutritionist, be guided by them because they will know your individual needs. If you find you cannot take supplements at the suggested dosages build up to the full dosage slowly or take them two or three times a week instead of every day if that is all you can manage. Remember that supplements should be regarded as a medicine to correct deficiencies and as such should be taken as a course and not indefinitely unless this has been advised by your doctor or nutritionist. Follow the instructions on the bottle carefully and keep them out of the reach of children.

Recommended supplements
by Penny Davenport

The supplement list recommended to combat candida seems endless, so I have singled out those below which I feel are the most important.

Vitamins

Vitamin A

As beta carotene, 25,00 ius or 15mg in good-quality supplements – this is the same amount.

B complex

Single B vitamins should always be taken with the complex to ensure balance.

- Vitamin B5 500mg: Important for combating stress.
- Biotin 800mcg: Prevents the yeast from becoming invasive, often comes with folic acid.

Vitamin C

3–5g, as a sustained release formula, or in small divided doses; anti-viral and immune boosting.

Minerals

Zinc 15–50mg

Elemental form, the dose on the label is often higher so check; for immune function.

Selenium 200mcg

Inhibits free radical damage.

Kelp 2–6 daily

All essential trace minerals; excellent for balancing the thyroid gland, which often contributes to a low immune system.

Magnesium 200mg

Taken in the morning, helps muscle ache and fatigue.

Probiotics

As well as bifido bacteria and acidophilus, lactobacillus salivarius is newly available; it digests protein molecules that have not been completely digested, a common cause of autotoxicity.

Digestive enzymes

Take 1–2 with each meal, or as needed. Incompletely digested food causes many problems. There are a variety of vegetarian formulations, and these are often preferred to the animal type; some are in vegetable gelatin.

Anti-parasitics

- Grapefruit seed concentrated extract. Many candida sufferers are found to have parasites.
- Frozen castor oil capsules.

Herbs

Garlic

Highly anti-fungal and promotes the growth of probiotic organisms.

Echinacea

Stimulates production of white blood cells.

Combinations

- Artemesia, barberry, pulsatilla and zingiber with grapefruit extract, are antibiotic, anti-fungal and anti-parasitic.
- Chinese herbs like shizandra, acanthopanax and astragalus boost immunity.

Pau d'Arco tea

Boosts the immune system, and strongly anti-fungal.

Essential fatty acids

Gamma linoleic acid and evening primrose oil 1–4g daily. Essential to produce balanced hormones, prostaglandins; one function is to keep yeast cells at bay, and to stimulate the immunity gland, the thymus, to produce T-cells.

If you are on a limited income, you must stick to the diet first. It is not expensive – think what you would save on your normal shopping bill: no bread, biscuits, cakes, tea, coffee, sweet drinks, no dairy products, not to mention sweets and chocolate, all of which leaves a lot of room for a variety of vegetables. Never go hungry, eat small meals regularly, and drinking water is important.

As supplements are expensive it is important to know which ones to choose and ways of being economical. Vitamin C is essential; the powder is the cheapest, especially as plain ascorbic acid. Buffered with minerals, it costs a little extra. Herbs are always economical and making a tisane is simple. Capsules and tablets cost more, but generally less than £10 for a three to four weeks' supply. As they boost the immune system and are anti-fungal, and in some cases anti-parasitic as well, the new combinations can be useful. With probiotics try the cheaper ones first to see if they work for you, but sometimes it makes more sense to take less of a quality concentrated form, but find the one that works for you.

Garlic is important, so eat as much as you can, but if this is socially impossible there are odourless varieties, but as they are highly concentrated they are more costly. A good all-round food concentrate that gives a wide range of essential nutrients is a fresh water algae called Chlorella. Many sympathetic practitioners dispense supplies in weekly packs, so it is always worth asking. If you cannot find one or your local health shop does not stock the items you want, there are excellent mail order companies who also specialize in giving advice (see Useful addresses).

Penny Davenport, a member of the Register of Nutritional Therapists, has worked as a nutritional adviser for more than 20 years. She gives personal and telephone consultations specializing in candida and detoxification problems.

Diet neurosis

Practitioners helping people with candida and allergy problems have increasingly become aware of what I have called 'candida/allergy diet neurosis'. Some people (even those under medical supervision) become so obsessed by what they can't eat that the diet becomes very narrow. They become malnourished and this affects the immune and nervous systems, with the result that there have been hospital admissions for nervous breakdowns and anorexia.

Relax, be balanced, have the odd treat, rotate your foods, watch your weight and above all understand that dietary adjustments are a temporary medicine to clean the digestive tract and help your immune system. What is the point of ending up with a pristine digestive tract if you have endangered your health in other ways?

11

Looking after yourself

Taking care of your general health is a vital part of the anti-candida programme. Stimulating the circulation and lymphatic system by exercise and getting plenty of fresh air and daylight should be taken very seriously. Early nights are also essential.

Exercise

Exercise is an important part of recovery from most conditions but it is often hard to convince people of this. They seem to think that because they feel low they should be as inactive as possible. If you do not have a fever, inflamed muscles, or any condition likely to be adversely affected by exercise, such as ME (check with your doctor if you are unsure), then move; you will delay your recovery if you don't.

It would be unwise to start vigorous activities if you have been sitting around for months. Build up the amount of exercise slowly. You will see below why it is so important.

Inactivity affects the circulation and consequently organic function. For example, the digestion becomes sluggish; this causes constipation. Muscles are also affected, not only by lack of nourishment, but also by a build-up of crystals that are formed from the waste products of digestion. This can cause generalized aches and pains and local tender spots. If you don't move, the crystals cannot be dispersed. Tension also locks these crystals into the muscles; a build-up in the shoulder area can be very painful and, in turn, cause you to move less.

If you do not move the muscles of the neck and shoulders, you restrict the blood supply to the head and give yourself endless problems. You need to ask yourself how much you are holding yourself back by sitting long hours in a car, at a desk or even watching television without moving. The brain can become sluggish, too, and when full circulation is restored symptoms of anxiety and depression can be dramatically relieved. Building simple stretching exercises into your daily life or a brisk walk in your lunchtime break take little time and can be a start, but you have to make more time for exercise if you really want to feel the benefits.

Fluid retention

The lymphatic system has been described so you will understand the importance of movement for the lymph fluid to be sent around the body.

Building movement into daily living

Be aware of how you are moving when you are walking. Could you lengthen your stride and stretch the muscles more?

Could you make an effort to get out of the car more frequently if you have to drive a lot? If you take several short walks, stretching your legs and swinging your arms, you will be less tired at the end of the day.

Exercise can be incorporated into housework. If you stop in the middle of your ironing and lie on the floor and 'bicycle' for a few minutes you will be sending the lymph fluid in the right direction – towards the shoulders. Your feet will ache less too.

Sitting at a computer for hours puts a terrible strain on the body. Take as many breaks as you can. Contracting the muscles of the feet, thighs and buttocks also helps if you can't leave your seat too much.

I'm too tired to exercise

Even if you have to stay in bed for some reason you can still help to circulate the lymph by gently squeezing each group of muscles in turn, and rotating the ankles and wrists. Massage can also be very helpful.

Aerobic exercise

Aerobic exercise is, by definition, exercise that utilizes the long, smooth muscles of the upper legs and arms. This muscle pumps blood (and lymphatic fluid) to the heart and liver, and to the lungs for cleansing and oxygenating, thereby boosting the immune system by encouraging regeneration and white blood cell replacement. Aerobic exercise also stimulates the production of serotonin, a sleep precursor, and endorphins, which are pleasure-giving and pain-relieving. It promotes sleep because muscle growth and cell replacement is a result of exercise, but can only take place during sleep. It strengthens the muscles of the heart and increases the capacity of the lungs.

For aerobic exercise to be effective, it needs to be done for 20 minutes, three times a week, at a pace that makes you breathe deeply and hard, but not out of breath. A target heart-rate range must be sustained for 20 minutes. It should be an effort, but not exhausting. Swimming, walking, gentle jogging, running, cycling, step and aerobic classes are all examples of aerobic exercise.

Water therapies

The skin, in effect, is the largest organ in the body. While the digestive tract and the kidneys are the main organs of excretion the skin also has a very important part to play; it is a great deal more useful than just a waterproof covering that stops us falling apart. If it is kept healthy it can be a wonderful waste-disposal system. It covers such a large area it is worth getting it to work for you.

A fever is nature's way of helping us to lose toxins through the skin. You can stimulate sweating with some water therapies. Steam baths, saunas and jacuzzis encourage detoxification. Exercises in water or swimming also stimulate the lymphatic system and rid the body of toxins.

Caution: Consult your doctor before using water treatments if you have heart trouble, raised blood pressure, diabetes, epilepsy or have any condition that might be aggravated by extremes of temperature. If you are on medication, particularly tranquillizers, it is also advisable to check with your doctor.

Sea bathing

The tonic effect of sea bathing is well known but perhaps it is less well known that even walking ankle deep in the sea boosts circulation and can be very soothing for the nervous system. Tension can be discharged through the soles of the feet as they are massaged by the sand – rather like the effect of reflexology.

Hydrotherapy

Hydrotherapy has been used in spas for thousands of years. During the past hundred years the popularity of hydrotherapy has waned and people have turned away from natural healing methods toward drugs, sometimes with disastrous results. Those who have sought water treatments have often been regarded as cranks. Public opinion could, however, be influenced by the work of Professor Vijay Kakkar, of the Thrombosis Research Institute in London.

Cold baths (TRHT)

Professor Kakkar's research has shown that thermo-regulatory hydro-therapy (TRHT) strengthens the immune system, boosts testosterone in men and oestrogen in women (this could help menopausal symptoms), increases the circulation, helps asthma and could prevent throm-bosis. A research programme was carried out at the Institute on 5,000 volunteers. Professor Kakkar stated: 'We are putting a scientific sense into something that is widely practised. This is for the benefit of the people. That is why I wanted to publish it now,' he said. 'But I would strongly urge those interested in this to adhere to the programme and follow the health warnings.'

Salt baths

Salt baths encourage detoxification and greatly help muscle and joint pains. Add three cupsful of sea salt or Epsom salts to a comfortably hot bath and lie in it for 20 minutes; add hot water as it cools. Drinking a pint of hot water with the juice of half a lemon and a teaspoonful of honey, or peppermint tea, while you soak will further encourage sweating. An ice-pack or cold flannel on the forehead might make you feel more comfortable.

Afterwards, wrap up in warm towels or a cotton sheet and get into a warm bed and you should perspire freely and sleep well. If you take a bath during the day finish with a cold shower and rest for half an hour. You could do this three times weekly.

Foot baths

You could have a foot bath while reading or watching the television. It helps to stimulate the circulation and ease aching feet. Use bowls of hot and cold water alternately, staying two minutes in each for a total of about 20 minutes. You could add one cup of salt or half a cup of Epsom salts to the hot water and an ice pack to the cold. When you have finished, wrap the feet in a towel and rest.

Swimming

Swimming stimulates the immune system and has been shown to elevate mood. Allergy sufferers may be affected by chlorinated water in swimming pools.

Skin brushing

For people who hate exercise, this is a good way to stimulate the lymphatic system. It involves brushing all over with a natural bristle brush for about ten minutes before your shower or bath. Start with the soles of the feet and work on all areas except broken skin, the face, neck and breasts. It can be boring but the results are worth it. In addition to eliminating toxins, because circulation is increased, it will also improve the texture of your skin. Skin brushes are widely available from chemists; or you might have an old hairbrush that would do the job, but wash it carefully first.

Light, sun, air

Daylight is necessary for normal brain functioning and for the regulation of the sleep–wake cycle; staying indoors when you are depressed or ill can only compound your problems. Even if you are severely agoraphobic you could sit at an open window without your glasses; do this for a minimum of 20 minutes daily in the brightest part of the day.

Sunlight kills bacteria and fungus on the skin. Short exposure to ultraviolet light, either from the sun or a sun bed can be of great benefit to fungal skin infections. Baking in the sun for hours or overdoing sun bed treatments ages the skin and can lead to skin cancer. Frequent exposure for short periods has other beneficial effects, including the production of vitamin D. We also look healthier after a little sun and this increases feelings of well-being.

Exposure to fresh air also kills fungus. Unless they actually have chest problems, it is often difficult to convince people of the benefits of good breathing habits, and even harder to impress upon them the dangers of continually filling the lungs with stale air. Candida sufferers should avoid being in dank, mouldy places such as cellars and damp rooms and going out when the weather is warm and moist. At such times the air is laden with fungal spores. They should, as has been said in Chapter 6 on allergies, avoid paint fumes, being near photocopiers and other chemical pollutants.

Complementary therapies

A brief mention is all that is possible here because of space. All the well-known therapies, such as acupuncture, homoeopathy, osteopathy, massage and reflexology have helped some people although you might have to try a few before you find the right one for you.

Kinesiology

This has special mention because it can do so much. It is a painless muscle-testing technique where the answers come from your own body. Pathogens can be detected, organs under strain are identified, vitamin and mineral deficiencies can be found and products your body will benefit from can be tested. The treatment changes the body energies so that they are balanced and can deal with the problems found. Some kinesiologists find it useful to see what medications and supplements you are taking, and ask you to prepare a list of questions about your health that you would like answered.

For information see the websites <www.hk4health.co.uk> (UK) and <www.subtlenergy.com> (USA).

Treatment for CFS/ME: The Phil Parker Lightning Process

The Phil Parker Lightning Process training programme has successfully helped hundreds of chronically ill people to break out from the spiral of illness, and so regain control over their lives. It claims high success rates (over 90 per cent) and dramatic recovery from symptoms of the range of disorders that include ME, CFS, post-viral syndrome (PVS) and Lyme disease.

It has also created a breakthrough in many areas of health care where nothing else seems to work, including anxiety and panic attacks, obsessive-compulsive disorder (OCD), depression, low self-esteem, self-doubt, guilt and a wide range of physical issues.

The programme was designed by Phil Parker DO, drawing from his training as an osteopath, hypnotherapist, NLP master and life coach, and teaches a whole new set of tools and ways of thinking that allow people not only to regain their health but also to be back in charge of their life again. For more details, visit <www.lightningprocess.com> or <info@lightningprocess.com>.

Electrical pollution

The immune system can be affected by working environments contaminated by low-level radiation from electrical equipment and from an overload of positive ions. If ventilation is poor, and we walk on synthetic carpets, wear synthetic clothes and are surrounded by plastic furniture, we are unlikely to feel good at the end of the day. In cities, stale air can be trapped between tall buildings. Electrically polluted air can be the cause not only of respiratory problems but also of headaches, irritability, digestive problems and depression.

Particles in the air around us, ions, are electrically charged, positive and negative. There should be a balance between the two. We breathe in these particles and absorb them through the skin. If the air is overloaded with positively charged particles it can have a powerful effect on the nervous system. The brain overproduces a chemical called serotonin and the effects of this can include nasal congestion, lethargy, feeling sticky (not the same feeling as being too hot) and swollen. The oppressive feeling before an electrical storm best describes this, a restless feeling, being 'under the weather'.

Negative ions have a tonic effect on the nervous system and reduce histamine levels in the blood. As any allergy sufferer knows, histamine is strongly associated with unpleasant feelings. The benefits of negative ionization are becoming widely known not only for cleaning the air, killing bacteria and viruses, but also as a treatment for asthma, bronchitis, migraine, burns, scalds and wounds. Candida sufferers, particularly if they have allergies, would do well to buy an ionizer to use in the bedroom. They are also available for use in a car and can be found in most department stores. After a thunderstorm the air is negatively charged; it smells fresh and we experience 'the calm after the storm', our energy returns and our mood improves. The air by the sea, waterfalls and flowing water, even by the shower, is also negatively charged and can produce a feeling of well-being. Some people are more affected by this than others, in the same way that some people are irritable and restless when the moon is full and others do not notice it. At full moon, the positively charged layer of the ionosphere, air and particles that absorb harmful radiation from the sun, is pushed nearer the earth, thus increasing the number of positive ions in the air we breathe.

You cannot overdo negative ions; there is no maximum dosage, you can breathe in as many as you like. Some people have ionizers in every room. If you have one in your sitting-room don't forget to put it by your bed at night where it will help you to have a restful night.

The state of the electromagnetic field

We are electrical beings: our hearts, brains, muscles and nerves all produce a subtle form of electricity and this discharges around our bodies and forms an electromagnetic field. All living things are surrounded by this field. It can be imagined as a glow around the body similar to that which surrounds an electric light bulb, although it is not just white but contains many colours. These can be seen clearly in photographs where a GDV (gas discharge visualization) camera has been used. In the 1930s in Russia, Kirlian photography clearly showed this field. It also showed that a leaf torn in half still showed the full electrical field.

The influence on the whole being – body, mind and soul – of the electromagnetic field (also known as an 'aura') is dismissed by many scientists and considered merely to be mystical nonsense. This is unfortunate since some experts believe that disease manifests in the electromagnetic field before physical symptoms appear. This can be demonstrated by Kirlian photography.

One of the first people to study what he called the 'L-fields' or the 'fields of life' and how they affect health, was Harold Saxon Burr, of Yale University Medical School.

Dr Robert O. Becker, co-author of *The Body Electric* (1998), and a leading researcher on electromagnetic pollution, believes that human-made electromagnetic fields from power lines and electrical appliances can cause depression, a depressed immune system and other health problems. His studies and those of others have shown higher incidences of depression, suicide and increased cancer risks near pylons. Working on the electromagnetic field could be the medicine of the future, the prevention and treatment of illness through balancing areas of low energy. This knowledge is not new, and similarities can be found in ancient forms of healing.

The East has acknowledged this energy for thousands of years: prana (life force), the meridians (paths of this energy down the body) and the chackras (seven main collections or 'power houses' down the centre of the body), are terms used in mainstream medicine. In the western world the same terms are well known in acupuncture and other complementary therapies.

Therapeutic touch

Because of the work of American nurse Dolores Krieger, a technique that clears and energizes the electromagnetic field is taught in some nursing schools; it is known as therapeutic touch. She describes this in her book *The Therapeutic Touch: How To Use Your Hands to Help or to Heal*. Janet Macrae, one of Dolores Krieger's students, has written a simple book that anyone can use, called *Therapeutic Touch: A Practical Guide*, published by Kopf. Do not worry if you do not feel the different qualities of the energies she describes when you are working either on yourself or other people: what you feel is what you feel; don't try to fit that into the experience of someone else. Your hands are unique.

Can I feel my own electrical field?

Only 1 per cent of people can't, so try it. You might need a few attempts before you can be sure, but the more you practise, the more sensitive your hands will become. There are several ways to build up the energy in your hands before you use them. Here is a simple one I saw in a Julie Soskin workshop. Breathe in slowly and visualize yourself being filled with Universal Energy, prana, ch'i or whatever you wish to call it.

Increasing the energy between your hands

1 Hold your arms out in front of you, raising one about a foot above the other.
2 Clench and release the fists rapidly for about 15 seconds.
3 Lower the raised hand and raise the other; repeat the fist clenching and releasing.
4 Keeping the arms out in front; repeat 2 and 3.
5 Relax the shoulders; point the fingers upwards as if you were going to clap. Make a 'concertina' movement with the hands in and out, just a few inches but do not bring the palms into contact.

You will feel a resistance or a feeling of pressure, heat or tingling between your hands. Some people say that they feel as if there is foam rubber between their palms, others describe feelings of tingling, throbbing or pulling.

Using your hands to clear the electromagnetic field

Now that your hands are energized you can use them to clear positive ions from your immediate environment, relieve headaches and nasal congestion, increase relaxation, and ease discomfort in muscles and joints.

1 Rub your feet and massage under the arch for about a minute. If your feet are very tense take a little longer over it, then place them flat on the floor if sitting.
2 Sit relaxed or lie on the floor or bed; slow down your breathing.
3 Close your eyes and imagine yourself totally well and peaceful. If you cannot get this image, give yourself the command, 'I am totally well and peaceful', and imagine a pure white light is entering your head, filling your body and coming out from your fingers and palms. Reach up beyond your head and stroke about three to four inches above your body just as though you were touching it; down over your face, neck, chest and abdomen, and then sweep the hands to either side of the body. This is important because you need to take the congestion clear of your body. You will feel prickling or heat in your hands as you pick up congestion. You can just flick this off as though you are shaking water from your hands.
4 Continue stroking for about ten minutes or until your arms feel tired.
5 Now, still imagining you are filled with white light and seeing it coming from your hands, hold them over your abdomen and imagine your digestive tract and all your internal organs becoming healthy and vitalized.

Increasing energy in selected areas

In this part of the exercise you are sending energy to an area of discomfort, perhaps an aching knee or bloated abdomen. You may feel heat or cold and possibly rumblings in your gut. Don't be surprised if it makes loud noises. This is just a sign that you are relaxing. As you practise this you will get a feeling of being 'finished'. That is the only way to describe the sensation of an area having taken enough energy. You might also have noticed your nose feeling less congested or your sinuses making popping noises when you were working around your head. You can transfer energy in the same way to any aching muscles or joints that you can reach. Clearing congestion from the field also helps to cool a fever, ease itching and reduce swelling.

Many people get very enthusiastic about therapeutic touch and are keen to use it to help others. This is certainly to be encouraged but not before you are well and have learned more about it. There are people who teach this technique, which is sometimes called 'auric massage'.

Aqua Detox

Aqua Detox is a welcome, exciting new alternative therapy for detoxifying the body and restoring its natural healing energy levels. It balances the electromagnetic field of the body, or aura (described above). Another name for this is the bio-energetic system of the body. This essential part of the human organism is largely ignored by modern medicine.

The Aqua Detox machine

The Aqua Detox machine is becoming the world leader in body detoxification. It is a relatively new treatment that has been in use for only a few years. The machine looks like a footbath. The feet are immersed in water through which a very low voltage electrical current is passed. A unit called an 'array' creates a flow of electrons that changes the water to the same bio-energetic field as the person having the treatment. This allows positive and negative ions to travel through the body and stimulates the body through the meridians. This detoxifies the body and organs and has a positive effect on the microcirculation of the body. The body is rebalanced enabling better functioning of the organs.

Since there are more than 2,000 pores on the bottom of each foot, the water can be seen very quickly to change colour (orange, green or even black) due to the toxins leaving the body. Fat globules often appear on the surface of the water, which by the end of the half-hour treatment often smells unpleasant. The machine can be safely used by people of all ages, except during pregnancy and lactation and for people with pacemakers.

In *Cam*, the magazine for complementary and alternative medicine professionals (September 2005), Dr Sanjay Chaudhuri implemented a study which accurately assesses the Aqua Detox machine's effect on human physiology. Dr Chaudhuri concluded that overall the scientific results were impressive.

For more information visit <www.aquadetoxusa.com>.

Where can I get this treatment?

Because this treatment has been proven to help so many conditions it is hoped that one day it will be available within the NHS. Until then you'll need to find an alternative practitioner using Aqua Detox (see Useful addresses for a therapist in your area).

You must inform your therapist of any medication you are on. It is essential to drink lots of warm water for several days after the treatment. Your therapist will guide you on that. If your fluid intake is normally low it would make sense to increase it before the treatment. If your doctor has put you on restricted fluids, seek his or her advice before treatment.

There have been a few reports of side effects after treatment, such as headache and fatigue. Most people seem to feel fine, but when using any method to rid the body of toxins, even a change of diet, it is not unusual to experience aching limbs, lack of energy, loss of appetite and abdominal bloating. There can also be an emotional release, feeling a bit 'down' irritable or weepy. These feelings do not last. Take as much rest as you can and keep on drinking the water!

Eat sensibly

While on an anti-candida programme is not the time to embark on drastic slimming or cleansing diets. That does not mean eating junk foods either; be sensible and ensure that you have adequate protein. If you are underweight or your appetite is poor, take high-protein drinks.

The preceding chapter gave some useful healthy eating information and diets for anti-candida. Check that you are not anaemic and consider taking some of the supplements mentioned.

Chlorella is a supplement described by Dr Bernard Jensen, an internationally renowned nutritionist, as the 'gem of the Orient'. It balances the body chemistry, boosts the immune system and contains a wide range of vitamins, minerals and trace elements. It is tolerated well by most people because it is not stimulating and is easily digested.

The inner child, the spirit

This might appear to be a strange conclusion to a book on a parasitic yeast, but since I believe that total health is dependent on the harmony of body, mind and spirit, I felt the need to include, with humility, the little I have learned in my own emotional and spiritual struggle.

Parasitic emotions

Negative feelings about ourselves, lack of self-worth, lack of self-love, anger, failure to see our place in the world, and fears, particularly the fear of the death of our physical bodies, can continually eat away at our life force, preventing us living in the here and now, and disrupting our lives as much as yeast overgrowths in the gut, or any other physical problem.

Where do these feelings come from and why do we hang on to them? They come from our life experience (beginning prenatally), and we are often reluctant to give them up because in order to do this they have to be confronted. Most of us shy away from this out of fear, or we lack the insight to see that these suppressed emotions are causing us problems. We use tension, hyperventilation (over-breathing), physical illness, addictions to alcohol, drugs, sleep, power, work, TV, sport, gambling, searching for relationships, money, even compulsive talking and use of the telephone – any number of mechanisms – to contain the fear and emptiness of the inner child, thus building up the wall of neurosis (see my book *Coping with Anxiety and Depression*, published by Sheldon Press, 1996 and *Healing Your Aloneness*, by Erika J. Chopich and Margaret Paul, 1990).

Neurosis should not be used as a put-down word to describe what we consider odd behaviour in someone else; it simply means a reaction to trapped pain, an inner child, and consequently a soul, or whatever you may call your higher self, longing to be acknowledged, loved and brought together to make a whole person, a person who is centred, peaceful with yourself, your creator, and the world about you.

How can I love myself?

First, wake up, be open to the possibility that you are not meeting your needs. Find a counsellor, psychotherapist or even a friend to support you while you explore the answers to these questions.

Questions to ask yourself:

- Am I crying inside?
- Am I lonely, even in company?
- Am I using mechanisms like hyperventilation and addiction to alcohol?
- Am I judgemental?
- Do I continually criticize the behaviour of others?
- Do I blame others, my life circumstances, the world, for my feelings?
- Am I always looking for a tomorrow that never comes?
- Do I continually look to others for approval?
- Have I taken on board the negative feelings that people from my past and present – mother/father/siblings/teachers/employers/ partners – have about me?
- Do I feel their feelings about me to be unjust and untrue and yet reinforce their accusations by refusing to give them up?
- Am I afraid?
- Am I too afraid of fear itself to face why I am afraid?
- Am I afraid to express anger?
- Does my anger come out in inappropriate places – on the people I know will take my anger and still love me, or on strangers where I do not risk losing love?
- Am I afraid to love – even myself?
- Am I puzzled by my behaviour towards others; is it how I really want to behave?
- Do I feel totally unlovable?

Realize that self-love takes a great deal of practice and be aware that it is very different from narcissism and selfishness. M. Scott Peck in his book *The Road Less Travelled* (1990) covers this subject with wisdom and love.

Useful addresses

Abbey Brook Cactus Nursery
Old Hackney Lane
Darley Dale
Matlock
Derbyshire DE45 2QJ
Tel.: 01629 580306
Suppliers of *cactus peruvianus*, which is used to absorb low-level radiation.

Academy of Systematic Kinesiology
16 Iris Road
West Ewell
Epsom, Surrey KT19 9NH
Tel.: 020 8391 5988 (Tuesdays, Wednesdays, Fridays)
Website: www.kinesiology.co.uk

Action Against Allergy (AAA)
PO Box 278
Twickenham
Middlesex TW1 4QQ
Tel.: 020 8892 4949/2711
Website: www.actionagainstallergy.co.uk
AAA provides an information service on all aspects of allergy and allergy-related illness, which is free to everyone. Supporting members get a newsletter three times a year. AAA can supply the names and addresses of specialist allergy doctors. It also runs a talk-line network which puts sufferers in touch with others through the NHS and itself initiates and supports research. Please enclose s.a.e. (9 in. x 6 in.) for further information.

Action for ME
Third Floor, Canningford House
38 Victoria Street
Bristol BS1 6BY
Tel.: 0117 9279551 or Lo-call 0845 123 2380
Website: www.afme.org.uk

Allergy Testing (North-East Area)
Hazel White-Cooper
Homeopathic Practitioner
18 Wilmington Close
Tudor Grange
Kenton Bank Foot
Newcastle-upon-Tyne NE3 2SF
Tel.: 0191 286 5053
Specializes in allergy testing. If writing for details please enclose s.a.e.

Association and Register of Colonic Hydrotherapists (ARCH)
Tel.: 0870 241 6567
Website: www.colonic-association.org

BioCare Ltd
Lakeside
180 Lifford Lane
Birmingham B30 3NU
Tel.: 0121 433 3727
Website: www.biocare.co.uk
Wide range of nutritional supplements for candida control and allergies,
including probiotics, GLA, Mycropryl and children's formula.

Borrelia/ME
See **Wright, Dr Andrew**

British Holistic Medical Association
PO Box 371
Bridgwater
Somerset TA6 9BG
Tel.: 01278 722000
Website: www.bhma.org.uk

British Institute for Allergy and Environmental Therapy
Ffynnonwen
Llangwyryfon
Aberystwyth
Ceredigion SY23 4EY
Tel.: 01974 241376
Website: www.allergy.org.uk

British Society for Allergy, Environmental and Nutritional Medicine
PO Box 7
Knighton
Powys LD7 1WT
Information Line 0906 3020010
Website: www.bsaenm.org

Colonic International Association
See **Guild of Colonic Hydrotherapists**

Council for Information on Tranquillisers and Antidepressants (CITA)
The JDI Centre
3–11 Mersey View
Waterloo
Liverpool L22 6QA
Tel.: 0151 932 0102, 10 a.m. to 1 p.m., Monday to Friday
Website: www.citawithdrawal.org.uk

Edmundson, Elizabeth
18 Wilmington Close
Tudor Grange
Kenton Bank Foot
Newcastle upon Tyne NE3 2SF
Tel.: 0191 286 5053
Homoeopathic practitioner specializing in candida treatment. Please send s.a.e. for details.

G & G Food Supplies Ltd
Vitality House
2–3 Imberhorne Way
East Grinstead
West Sussex RH19 1RL
Tel.: 01342 312811
Website: www.gandginfo.com

Guild of Colonic Hydrotherapists
16 Drummond Ride
Tring
Herts HP23 5DE
Tel.: 01442 827687
Website: www.colonic-association.com

Habgood, Jackie (health practitioner)
40 Priors Hill
Wroughton
Swindon SN4 0RW
Tel.: 01793 813 493

Health Plus Ltd
Dolphin House
Unit 27, Cradle Hill Industrial Estate
Seaford
East Sussex BN25 3JE
Tel.: 01323 872277
Suppliers of the Cantrol Pack of supplements

Higher Nature
Burwash Common
East Sussex TN19 7LX
Tel.: 01435 884668 (general); 01435 884572 (customer services, 9 a.m. to 5 p.m., Monday to Friday)
Website: www.highernature.co.uk
Email (for general enquiries): info@higher-nature.co.uk
Email (for advice): nutrition@higher-nature.co.uk
Dedicated to providing a comprehensive nutritional service. Higher Nature offers a reliable service for candida/allergy testing. They make regular contributions of supplements and money to refugees and those in nutritional need.

Hyperactive Children's Support Group
Dept. W,
71 Whyke Lane
Chichester
West Sussex PO19 7PD

IBS and Gut Disorder Centre
C/o Michael Franklin
Tel.: 0845 4546 0944
Website: www.ibs-solutions.co.uk
Trained nutritionist with a special interest in chronic fatigue syndrome, candida and allergies.

IBS Network
Unit 5
53 Mowbray Street
Sheffield S3 8EN
Tel.: 0114 272 3253
Website: www.ibsnetwork.org.uk
Run by IBS (Irritable Bowel Syndrome) sufferers for people affected by IBS. It offers a quarterly newsletter, *Gut Reaction*, self-help groups, and a 'Can't wait' card. Membership costs £3–£6 p.a. depending on income. For further information send s.a.e.

International Federation of Aromatherapists
82 Chiswick High Road
London W4 1PP
Tel.: 020 8742 2605 (10 a.m. to 4 p.m., Monday to Friday)

Larkhall Green Farm
225 Putney Bridge Road
London SW15
Tel. 020 8874 1130

LifeTools (Relaxation aids)
12 Tilbury Close
Caversham
Reading
Berkshire RG4 5JF
Tel.: 01189 483444
Website: lifetools.com
Email: sales@lifetools.com
This firm produces electronic medical machines which work with two ear clips at the press of a button. The Alpha-Stim SCS reduces anxiety, improves concentration, lifts depression and aids sleep, and the Alpha-Stim 100 does the same and also treats pain via probes.

ME Association
4 Top Angel
Buckingham Industrial Park
Buckingham MK18 1TH
Tel.: 0870 444 1835
Website: www.meassociation.org.uk
Email: meconnect@meassociation.org.uk
Enclose s.a.e. if writing for information.

Midlands Asthma and Allergy Research Association (MAARA)
Kingsway House
Kingsway
Derby DE22 3HL
Tel.: 01332 362461
Website: www.maara.org

National Candida Society
PO Box 151
Orpington
Kent BR5 1UJ
Tel.: 01689 813039
Website: www.candida-society.org.uk

National Institute of Medical Herbalists
Elm House
54 Mary Arches Street
Exeter EX4 3PA
Tel.: 01392 426022
Website: www.nimh.org.uk
Email: nimh@ukexeter.freeserve.co.uk

New Nutrition
Penny Davenport
Woodland Road
Battle
East Sussex TN33 0LP
Tel.: 01424 773373
Website: www.battlehealthylivingclinic.co.uk
Email: info@healthylivingclinic
Experienced nutritionist can advise on nutrition, special diets, natural
health and skin care.

Nutrition Associates
Caltres House
Lysander Close
Clifton Moorgate
York YO30 4XB
Tel.: Lo-call 0845 166 2058
Medical practice: candida/allergy testing, nutritional profiles. Clinics are
also in London, Edinburgh and Windsor. Appointments are made through
the York clinic (Tel.: 01904 691591).

Nutriscene
Unit D, Altbarn Industrial Estate
Revenge Road
Lordswood
Chatham ME5 8UD
Tel.: 01634 861880
Supplies herbal combinations, including those to curb candida, detoxify
mercury from fillings and combat geopathic stress.

Optima Health and Nutrition
Concept House
Brackenbeck Road
Lidget Green
BD7 2LW
Tel.: 01274 526360
Sells organic products, including a tea-tree oil range under the brand
name 'Thursday Plantation'.

Perrin, Dr Raymond
The Perrin Clinic Manchester
11 St John Street
Manchester M3 4DW
Website: www.theperrinclinic.com
Email: drperrin@theperrinclinic.com
For people in the north-east of England, Anne Dand (remedial massage) and Crichton Dand (health kinesiology) are both trained in the Perrin treatment: phone 0191 258 7634.

The Radionic Association
Baerlein House
Goose Green
Deddington
Banbury
Oxfordshire OX15 0SZ
Tel.: 01869 338852
Website: www.radionic.co.uk
I can personally recommend (as can many of my clients and readers) radionics, a little-known alternative approach. It is useful in a wide variety of conditions. The Association can give details of practitioners in your area.

Tigon (GB) Ltd
Eden House
6 Edward Street
Anstey
Leics LE7 7PP
Tel.: 0116 2355020
Website: www.oliveleaf.co.uk

VegEPA
Igennus Ltd
St John's Innovation Centre
Cowley Road
Cambridge CB4 0WS
Tel.: 0845 1300 424
Website: www.vegepa.com
Also stocked by nutritionists.

Wright, Dr Andrew
Complete Hormone Clinic
Chronobiology Ltd
Dalton House
33 Leigh Road
Westhoughton
Bolton BL5 2JE
Tel.: 01942 819301 for appointment
Dr Wright is trained in orthodox and alternative medicine, and has a great interest in chronic fatigue syndrome and its links with borrelia (Lyme disease), allergies, candida and borreliosis.

Note for readers in the United States

The nutritional suppliers mentioned in this list are willing to mail their products to the USA. The same or similar products can be obtained from:

Interplexus Inc.
VitaminLife
15940 Redmond Way
Redmond
WA 98052
USA

North American Herb & Spice
Tel.: 1 800 243 5242 (General enquiries)
Website: www.p-73.com

Further reading

Becker, R. O. and Selden, G., *The Body Electric*. William Morrow, N.Y., 1998.

Chaitow, L., *Candida Albicans, The Non-Drug Approach to the Treatment of Candida Infection*. Thorsons, London, 2003.

Cheung, T., *How to Boost Your Immune System*. Sheldon Press, London, 2006.

Chopich, E. and Paul, M., *Healing Your Aloneness*. HarperSanFrancisco, Calif., 1990.

Clark, Dr Hulda, *The Cure For All Diseases*. New Century Press, Calif., 1995.

Craggs-Hinton, C., *Living with Fibromyalgia*. Sheldon Press, London, 2000.

Crook, Dr William G., *Chronic Fatigue Syndrome and the Yeast Connection*. Professional Books, Jackson, Tenn., 1992.

Crook, Dr William G., *The Yeast Connection Handbook: How Yeast Can Make You 'Sick All Over' and the Steps You Can Take to Regain Your Health*. Professional Books, Jackson, Tenn., 1999.

D'Adamo, Dr Peter J., *Eat Right for Your Type*. Century, London, 2001.*

Gazzola, A., *Living with Food Intolerance*. Sheldon Press, London, 2006.

Grant, D. and Joice, J., *Food Combining for Health*. Thorsons, London, 1984.

Kenton, L. and S., *Raw Energy*. Century Arrow, London, 2004.

Krieger, D., *The Therapeutic Touch: How to Use Your Hands to Help or to Heal*. Prentice-Hall, N.J., and IBG, 1992.

Macrae, J., *Therapeutic Touch: A Practical Guide*. Knopf, N.Y., 1988.

Marek, C. C., *The First Year: Fibromyalgia, the Patient-Expert Guide for the Newly Diagnosed*. Robinson, London, 2003.

Puri, Professor B., *Attention-Deficit Hyperactivity Disorder – A Natural Way to Treat ADHD*. Hammersmith Press, London, 2005.

Puri, Professor B., *Chronic Fatigue Syndrome – A Natural Way to Treat M.E.* Hammersmith Press, London, 2004.

Puri, Professor B. and Boyd, H., *The Natural Way to Beat Depression: The Groundbreaking Discovery of EPA to Change Your Life*. Hodder Mobius, London, 2004.

Scott Peck, M., *The Road Less Travelled*. Arrow, London, 1990.

Shoman, Mary J., *Living Well with Hypothyroidism: What Your Doctor Doesn't Tell You that You Need to Know*, Harper Collins, London, 2000.

Tolle, E., *The Power of Now*. Hodder & Stoughton, London, 2005.

Winderlin, C. with Sehnert, Dr K., *Candida Related Complex – What Your Doctor Might be Missing*. Taylor Trade Publishing, Lanham, Md., 1996.

*Eating according to your blood group is becoming very popular. It is recommended for all. ME patients have done well on this when a gluten-free diet has failed. It is mentioned for use with the Samen/Noni Extract for ME/Borrelia infection.

Index